ENERGY TYPES

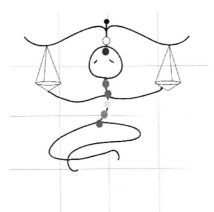

Personality,
Chakras
& Balance

Maureen Kelly

Dear Ellen,
Trust in The magic~
love, light healing
& balance...
maureen

Also by Maureen Kelly

Wine Types - Discover Your Inner Grape
Pet Types - Communing Heart To Heart

What a contribution! And a wonderful example of what can emerge if you follow your passions and intuition until all the pieces fit beautifully together as they have in this book.   This book is an obvious work of love by Maureen and in the application of her insights becomes an act of self-love on the part of the reader. Maureen goes beyond the limitations of "personality types" by meaningfully and powerfully blending the undeniable existence of our energy body. Her work raises the consciousness of what it means to be responsible, deliberate and loving towards ourselves as energy beings. An undeniable reality in these powerful times! Thank you, Maureen!!

Audrey Vitolins, of the *The Heart Brilliance Process*

Knowing our personality type is important but having tools to keep ourselves in balance is the icing on the cake. Maureen has done exactly this in her new book, *Energy Types*, in which she ties it all together with a toolkit full of yoga poses, breathing practices, affirmations and meditations for each personality type. It doesn't get any better.

Ellen Shea, Author of *I'm All Grown Up - Now What?*

The personality and chakra assessments found in *Energy Types* are right on! Maureen will open your eyes to your unique gifts and talents. I love her approach. She combines yoga poses, meditations and affirmations, giving the reader a complete toolkit to help nurture strengths, while supporting areas needing adjustment. You will feel grounded, focused and balanced.

Stacey Joiner, Author of *You Deserve the Royal Treatment*

Dedication

To my parents, Bud and Gwen Kelly
(ESTJ / ESFJ respectively),
for the stable, loving and
laughter-filled environment
they provided their ever quest-driven,
rescuer ENFJ daughter.
(I know there were times when
they shook their heads wondering,
"Where DID she come from?")
Endless gratitude and love...

TABLE OF CONTENTS

FOREWORD
Where East Meets West

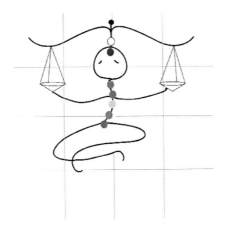

A VIEW FROM THE WEST...

There was a time when this thoroughly American, INTJ engineer, born and bred in a hard-working, blue-collar, Baptist home in a mostly white, South Jersey beach resort would have raised an eyebrow or two (or at least one large monobrow) at the notion of linking the Jung inspired "Type" genius of Isabel and Katharine with chants, chakras, yoga positions, and the lore of the East. But that was before my working in over forty countries, living with Montagnards in Vietnam, working with Hmungs in Laos, learning to respect the culture of Yemeni Arabs in Qatar, striding across the Serengeti with Massai warriors, and watching vultures participate in a Zoroastrian funeral at the top of the Tower of Silence in Mumbai, India.

Those of us who work with the MBTI® have become accustomed

in the last few years to looking at the links between what were at one time competing technologies and systems such as Keirsey's Temperament Theory, Gardiner's seven modalities of intelligence, the psychospiritual typology of the Enneagram, and the emerging science behind Emotional Intelligence. These systems of understanding the self and others, which at one time did not even receive a hearing at Type conferences, now almost dominate the breakout sessions at many international conferences. We have come to see how each can enhance our understanding of the other. As we increasingly work across borders and among cultures very different from our own, it is critical that we begin to appreciate the wisdom of others very different from ourselves.

We are relatively parochial learners in the West, and it has taken us a while to realize the truth behind novelist Anita Nim's admonition that "We [really] do not see things as they are. We see things as we are." Those of us reared in the Western world tend to see things from the perspective of a logical, cognitive, dialectical model. As a dominant iNtuitive (INTJ), I have mostly ignored the a-cognitive wisdom of the East for years. Jung would be displeased with me. While a Swiss-German by birth, Carl Gustav Jung was the first modern thinker to connect East with West. His desire that human beings recognize the connectivity of Body, Mind, and Spirit and the need for holism to become the complete human beings we are intended to become, lies at the heart of the connection between the MBTI® and Chakras.

What Maureen has done in this brief "ballet of creation" is to link the well-documented technology of the Myers-Briggs Type Indicator® with the wisdom of the East in very practical, easy to follow exercises. Without using technical language, she links Gardiner's modalities of cognitive intelligence, interpersonal intelligence, and intrapersonal intelligence (MBTI® and EQ) with bodily-kinesthetic intelligence.

I remember the first time I walked on African soil; it was like coming home. I had never been there before, but as I walked the trails and mingled with the tribes and the wildlife, it just felt right. Something whispered, "What took you so long? This is home."

As I review the Toolkit for the INTJ to regain balance and practice the meditations, affirmations, and Pranayama associated with Third Eye Chakra, Root Chakra, and Heart Chakra, it just feels right. Something seems to say, this is where you belong. This is the balance you need. What took you so long? I hope you have the same experience.

Be competent and be at peace.

William C. Jeffries, Author of *Still True to Type*
and CEO of Executive Strategies International, Inc.

A VIEW FROM THE EAST...

As we know, there are many paths that lead to holistic healing. In my experience, the path of the heart is the one to follow. *Energy Types* is a heart-felt inspiration that will take you on a journey of self- discovery.

Although my background is based in the ancient tradition of Ayurvedic healing, I was able to easily comprehend and apply the toolkit created by Maureen. For those of you unfamiliar with Ayurveda, it is the sister science of yoga and a comprehensive healing system that originated in India well over 5,000 years ago. This system includes not only nutrition, herbology, yoga asana, pranayama and meditation, but everything in our lives with which we interact. My teacher, Dr. Vasant Lad, summarizes this concept succinctly, "Ayurveda defines life as the conjunction of the body, mind and spirit found in Cosmic Consciousness and embracing all of Creation."

Ayurveda is based upon the laws of nature and the five elements. These elements of ether, air, fire, water and earth coalesce into unique patterns that make up each individual. There are three doshas or body/mind types that Ayurveda utilizes to restore equilibrium, whereas the MBTI® uses personality type. What I find fascinating is that the systems of both of these modalities enable people to gain a deeper understanding of their unique make up and with that knowledge the ability to heal themselves.

I appreciate that *Energy Types* resonates with the ancient truth that we, as unique individuals, need customized wellness plans to bring us back into balance. According to Ayurveda, everything, including us, comprises the five elements. What that means to me is that while each human being is entirely unique and never to be duplicated, every human does have natural tendencies that can either lead toward balance or imbalance ~ depending upon how we live our lives. At this point in the history of the world, it is challenging to maintain our essential connection with nature when, for many of us, the pace of our lives is very fast and often externally focused. *Energy Types* gives us an accessible, yet comprehensive doorway into a deeper understanding of the inner world of our chakras (vital energy points) and our mental functions. For thousands of years, Ayurveda has understood that each person has a preference for how they best receive information. It is refreshing to see that *Energy Types* offers an entire multimedia package that allows such variety: listening to the meditations, reading the text and using the cheerful yoga posture drawings to integrate the experience into one's own being.

It was very insightful to learn that according to my MBTI® results, I am an INFP. Knowing this, I was able to customize my practice and experiment with the Heart, Solar Plexus, and Root Chakra toolkits. I found it especially interesting that the balancing practices offered correspond perfectly with the Ayurvedic balancing recommendations for my body/mind type. The practices were not only enjoyable and fresh, but also effective. For instance, the Intentions, Affirmations and Earth Meditation for the root chakra were easy to incorporate as I worked toward becoming more grounded   I also like the fact that other chakras are included with which to experiment, as my requirements may change at different times.

According to one of the classic Ayurvedic texts, the Charaka samhita, "The Science of Life shall never attain finality. Therefore humility and relentless industry should characterize your endeavor and your approach to knowledge. The entire world consists of teachers for the wise and enemies for the fools. Therefore, knowledge, conducive to health, longevity, and excellence, should be received, assimilated and utilized with earnestness."

I hope each of you utilizes *Energy Types* fully in order to further understand and celebrate your uniqueness. Not only will these concepts enhance your experience of yourself, but will also build understanding and compassion for others.

Blissful healing,

Juliet Jivanti
Director of the Ayurvedic Health Center in Bellingham, Washington and creator of the DVD *"Ayurvedic Yoga: Yoga for Your Body Type"*

INTRODUCTION

How The Roads Converged

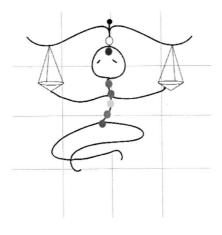

countless are the rivulets
running into this river of God.
choose your tributary wisely
where the stream is least impeded
as we joyfully flow together
into the ocean of oneness...

no matter the path we choose
we are all connected.
a continuous flow...
an evolving tapestry...
a ballet of creation...
where the dancers become the dance.
- Maureen

PERSONALITY + CHAKRAS = ENERGY TYPES

*W*ould our time on this planet be different if we were handed an instruction manual upon our arrival? "Welcome to Earth. Take a moment to read over the following guidelines to streamline and enhance your mortal experience and allow you to be the very best human you can be."

Well, I guess my aspirations in writing this book are to marry together the various modalities that I believe can assist us in living each day to the fullest and maybe ease some of the angst caused by the lack of having a manual for counsel.

When I was first introduced to the Myers- Briggs Type Indicator®, a Jungian-based personality assessment, it was a turning point in my life. I had just returned to the United States after spending nearly 10 years in Germany. (My American friends tell me that I 'missed the 80's'... odd perspective as this is based on my indifference to 'Who shot JR' and lack of knowledge as to who Mork & Mindy were...) Anyhow, my time in Europe included extensive travel and I had become fluent not only in German, but conversant as well in French, Italian and Spanish. That to me was quite representative of being an 'able communicator.'

Upon my re-entry to the U.S., however, where much to the chagrin of my poor husband I took to comparing EVERYTHING to 'how they did it in Europe,' I filled out my first MBTI® and a whole *new* world of communication was made available to me. I came to truly understand the concept of 'speaking the same language' and it didn't necessarily mean English, German or Italian. It went a whole lot deeper than that. (Hence the gaps experienced with fellow countrymen. Mork who?)

My fascination with these concepts and the love of what I was learning led me to complete my certification as a Myers-Briggs® consultant. Thanks to some wonderful teachers, (one in particular who graciously contributed to the foreword of this book) I went on to work with many businesses as well as individuals, sharing with them the valuable lessons this instrument had to offer.

Over time I expanded my use of typology to include comparing us to a varietal (*Wine Types - Discover Your Inner Grape*) as well as our communication styles with our 4-leggeds (*Pet Types - Communing Heart To Heart*). And while these undertakings were fun AND educational, I just knew there was a missing piece.

After all those years of 'analyzing' friends, pets and grapes (sometimes ad nauseum), I became certified as a yoga instructor. I began teaching what I call "Chakra Yoga" where we focused each week on a different energy field in our body. This included not only certain poses, but also breathing techniques and meditations that would further enhance whichever realm we were currently addressing. I was totally captivated by the whole concept of the energy 'swirling' within us.

And then it happened. It was as if a veil was lifted. THIS was the missing piece. **I became aware of the distinct correlation between our personalities and the realization that these leanings could cause an imbalance in our energy fields. Wow.**

What IS This All About?

In a time when so many are searching to determine a life's purpose or even just asking "Why the heck am I here?", the Myers-Briggs Type Indicator® offers a tangible roadmap in what can often prove to be a somewhat nebulous voyage. By getting answers to four key questions, we are presented with a prototype for embracing life's wonder: How do we perceive reality? How do we make our decisions? How are we energized? What characterizes our lifestyle? This instrument goes way beneath the surface and mines the gold found within each one of us. By offering solid principles to understand one's own strengths and vulnerabilities, as well as a blueprint for comprehending why other people behave the way they do, we gain priceless counsel!

It's All Energy...

Over the years when holding workshops or practicing individual consulting sessions, I would explain that we are a combination of nature and nurture; but I believed, as did Jung, that nature was the predominant factor. I would give examples of identical twins separated at birth having identical types or simple stories of families where children are being raised in the same manner but exhibiting very different likes, dislikes and modes of behavior. Yes, I would continue, environmental factors play a key role, but mainly in their fortification or weakening of a particular characteristic that in and of itself remained constant.

While I still maintain that nature is the predominant influence, a 'new' line of thought has also entered my awareness. I have in the past also used the terminology: "genetic vs environmental influence." However, considering our increased knowledge in the field of genetics, it personally no longer fits the mold to use this phraseology. I am definitely only skimming the surface here on a much, much deeper topic, but to explain it briefly, knowing now that genes actually have what could be referred to as an 'on/off' switch changes everything. For example, say from a health perspective that heart disease runs in your family. In times past we might then assume that YOU, therefore, have a proclivity for developing cardiac problems. But because THOUGHT is energy, by merely altering our way of thinking and changing our own expectations, we can indeed alter these once 'predictable' avenues of health or for that matter, behavior patterns. This is not only an amazing discovery, but an extremely liberating one!

So, given the latest developments within the more advanced and open medical communities regarding energy healing, the findings are not only fascinating, they are life-changing. The whole premise that we are indeed NOT the end product of our DNA's genetic makeup opens the door to an entirely new perspective in regards to taking control of our health. When we focus our intent on the preservation *or* the restitution of peak health within our body, we take ownership of the most precious gift we can possess, as optimum health - of body as well as spirit - is the precursor to peace of mind.

I'm Pickin' Up Good Vibrations...

So, how does all this tie in with the information found within these pages? The tapesty of these two arenas - personality and chakras - provides a springboard for balance, growth and manifestation of our life purpose in a healthy, vital environment. Through recognition and enhancement of our natural gifts, this information can be incorporated with our understanding of the energy fields within our physical and etheric body.

How To Get There From Here

We'll begin this journey by exploring the various personality characteristics from an individual perspective as well as how you 'mesh' with other personalities. Gaps in communication, be they internal (lack of personal direction) or external (friends, family, colleagues) can lead to confusion and distress. Unchecked, this upset can escalate and cause emotional as well as physical repercussions.

We will then move on to that magic that flows through each of us on an energetic plane and how we can tap into it on a more cognitive level. Through the various chakra 'toolkits' i.e. yoga poses, meditations, affirmations and mudras (seals or hand yoga) we can celebrate our strengths, nurture our souls, and restore balance when the scales are tipped. Maintaining a regular practice of yoga and meditation, especially with emphasis on our more susceptible areas can be akin to making deposits in our 'health bank account.'

If you are familiar with the movie "Man On Wire," a story of an amazing tight rope walker who performed some incredible feats, you will see that he held a long stick to aid him in maintaining his equilibrium. And he wasn't looking down... he was looking where he wanted to go. Think of these toolkits as our 'balance stick.'

Quieting our minds, becoming one with our heart and breath, and stretching our bodies will widen our own platform.

Oh, One More Thing...How to Read This Book

Okay, that last header either had you nodding your head, thinking, "Oh good. Directions." OR it had you muttering, "No one needs to tell me how to read a book. I'll do it how ever I please." With *that* in mind, you can read the following 'instructions' or completely ignore them.

Energy Types is divided into five categories that will offer you the following information:

1) *A discussion of the four personality preference pairs that make up the core of the MBTI®*

2) *An introduction and overview of the chakras (energy fields)*

3) *An overview of all 16 MBTI® personality types and references to the toolkits that will be most supportive of your Type*

4) *Chakra toolkits for each energy field*

5) *Taking AIM: Affirmation, Intention & Motion - Generic flows for every Type*

There are many wonderful books available that offer thought-provoking messages with the goal of bringing you to a place of understanding and personal peace. My hope with *Energy Types* is that it will give you tangible information, not only from an intellectual perspective, but from a physical standpoint as well. Where East meets West... bringing two worlds together in collaborative manifestation. Trust in the magic and see where it goes. Life is truly an adventure. Breathe it, embrace it, cherish it.

So fellow Earthlings, welcome to the world of *Energy Types*.

Wishing you love, light, healing & balance,
Maureen (ENFJ)

P.S. While this book was penned with my love of the human species in mind, portions of all proceeds from *Energy Types* will be directed to two of my favorite animal nonprofit organizations; this in support of beings who may not be heard as they attempt to communicate their needs. One of my deepest desires is to bridge that gap... because I truly believe our treatment of animals is representative of kindness overall.

ENERGY TYPES

CHAPTER 1

Our Preferences:
The Building Blocks of Personality

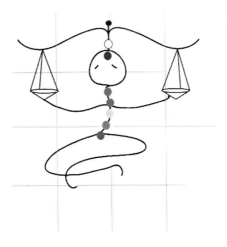

Your vision will become clear only
when when you look with your heart.

Who looks outside, dreams.
Who looks within, awakens.

- Carl Jung

The Fascinating World of Type

*W*hile we are all unique individuals, (some of us more so than others...ha ha) we are all indeed connected to one another as well. Becoming better acquainted with our own innate leanings can be a precious gift to ourselves. One of the beautiful 'side effects' of embracing this knowledge is that we become much more cognizant of why the other people in our lives behave (or misbehave depending on your viewpoint) the way they do. This awareness can open up pathways to communication that will greatly facilitate the flow of relationship in your life, which in turn will lead to smoother sailing in your OWN boat.

The stress that we hold in our bodies, which can lead to both emotional as well as physical imbalance, is often times due to a miscommunication in an interpersonal relationship. If this friction is suppressed (or possibly not even recognized yet on a conscious level) the consequences will eventually make themselves known.

We can liken the communication between personality types to a radio transmitter and receiver. If you want to hear rock n' roll oldies but you are tuned into a rap station, my bet is that you wont be hearing any Roy Orbison. The same proves true with our lines of communication. If you want to be understood, speaking the language of the party with whom you are engaging in conversation will make getting your point across a whole lot easier. This, of course, will be streamlined when you have an overall understanding of type and why folks conduct themselves the way they do.

I must digress here shortly to share with you an amusing story regarding interpersonal communication and how our lines can be crossed. Having lived in Germany for 'that missing decade' of the '80s, I became fluent in the language of the land. Sometimes, just for fun, I would 'teach' family or friends who came to visit a word or phrase of the day so that they could interact with the locals.

Well, some might call it cruel, but on more than one occasion I kind of 'slipped' when giving them the proper translation, in totally joyful anticipation of the reactions this would cause. One particular scenario comes to mind... My mom and dad had been visiting for a couple of weeks and they were set to head back to the states the following morning. My German landlords, Fritz and Margaret, had come by to share in drinking a schnaps and to bid them 'Auf Wiedersehen.' Fritz held his glass aloft and with true sincerity offered the following in German, "Bud, Gwen, wishing you safe travels, good health and all the best that life can offer. We hope to see you again." He then looked to me to translate. Well, who knows what evil demon grabbed hold of me, but this is what came out of my mouth. "Mom, Dad, one of the most cherished German traditions when folks visit from other countries, is to take a live chicken back home with you to honor your travels. Fritz would like to present you with one now." I did everything in my power to maintain a serious expression as I looked at Fritz in his solemn expectancy and at the horror on my parents' faces, before breaking out in reams of laughter. (Karlheinz, their teenage son who spoke a little bit of

English KNEW something was up when he heard the word 'chicken.') I did, then of course, pass on Fritz's heartfelt translation. But it was just too much fun to pass up. (I have many more similar stories. Funny how visiting friends stopped asking me to translate for them.)

It is obvious that there will be gaps in understanding when we are speaking two different languages, but folks, this happens when we are both speaking the SAME language as well. That is why the MBTI® is such a godsend in giving us a guideline to follow, not only to bring balance into our own lives, but to truly appreciate why others in our lives express themselves as they do.

WHAT IS *YOUR* PREFERENCE?

Let's begin by breaking down the four preference pairs that make up the MBTI® and explore them each in some detail. We will all have our own comfort zones, and hence the terminology "preference," but you will also most likely find that you relate to bits and pieces of the 'other side' as well.

EXTRAVERTS* (E) AND INTROVERTS (I):
What pumps you up?
Myers-Briggs® literature uses the terms extraversion and introversion as Jung first used them, and preserves the original spelling of extraversion.

For the time being, please disregard all former definitions of these two concepts because from the MBTI® perspective, it's a different ball game. Extraverts aren't necessarily blabbermouths (though I'm sure they are out there) and Introverts don't necessarily hide behind a book or a computer (and I'm sure that they exist as well.)

The bottom line when understanding this preference is **WHERE DO YOU GET YOUR ENERGY or from another perspective, WHAT CHARGES YOUR BATTERY?**

Extraverts tend to get pumped up when they are around other people, especially like-minded folks. Even if they are dragging a bit from a busy schedule or a long day, after mingling among colleagues and friends at a social gathering, they will most likely see their energy level escalate. The outer world of people and things charges their battery.

The Introvert, on the other hand, prefers alone time or the company of one or two close friends to regain their verve. Retreating to the quiet of their internal world or an intimate gathering will be a welcome boost to their spirit.

We all do need a balance of both, though, whether you are an Introvert *or* an Extravert. Extraverts still require their share of quiet time, though too much of it can be draining. Introverts do indeed need people, but too many for too long a time could prove exhausting.

There are distinct differences in the ways that Extraverts and Introverts express themselves. As an example, say that you have been unemployed for a rather lengthy amount of time and have recently applied for a position that could be referred to as your 'dream job.' One morning, the phone rings and it's the manager of human resources calling to let you know that they would like you to start work the following Monday.

If you are an Extravert, chances are, after hanging up the phone with your new employer and shrieking with joy, you will immediately - if not sooner - dial your best buddy, your partner/spouse, your shrink AND your mother-in-law (even if she drives you nuts) to relay your good news. Extraverts (E's) have a distinct need to share what transpires in their lives because it makes it *real* for them. Now depending on the strength of this particular preference, you may ONLY phone your best friend. But typically, the news will be passed along to someone.

Now, picture the Introvert in this same scenario. After completing the conversation with the HR department, your mode of reaction would most likely involve some silent moments of inner gratification followed by the eventual sharing of the news with your spouse/partner when they return home. If you are an EXTREME Introvert, you may not share your news with ANYONE. When the day comes that you begin your new job, people will just wonder where you are off to every day now after being home for such a long period of time.

Extraverts also tend to have a vocal thought process. They will get from point A to point B by talking their way there. If your introverted spouse asks you if you would like to go out for Mexican food, the response could possibly sound something like this: "Well, we were going to try and save some money and we have all of those leftovers in the frig. BUT we haven't had Mexican food in forever and that really sounds good. Okay!" (The Introvert has long ago begun shaking his/her head thinking, "Why can't he/she just say yes or no?")

In similar conversation scenarios, the Introvert will normally think things through internally. This may or may not lead to a vocalized conclusion which can, of course, lead to gaps in communication.

While the Extravert may share perhaps more information than necessary, the Introvert may fail to contribute *enough* information to clarify what could be an important issue.

I've always thought it's probably often an Introvert who has been given the job of translating the dialogue in subtitled movies. You know, when you HEAR, "aherlfuel foehreof eor dlmwighfe rofoehs bog eo fheor goe rheor bhe" and the translation underneath reads, "No." Gotta wonder...

DANGER ZONES

A danger zone when dealing with the Extravert could be their tendency towards thinking out loud. This may prove to be nothing more than idle rambling with no real action plan behind the dialogue. This can lead to confusion as those around them scratch their heads thinking, "But I KNOW I heard them say such and such...." SO, tips for dealing with Extraverts: CLARIFY, CLARIFY, CLARIFY. This is what I HEARD you say, but is it what you really MEAN?

Now the danger zone with the Introvert is just the opposite. An Introvert can actually hold an entire conversation WITH YOU in their head and truly believe that it took place. Let's say a conflict is brewing. It might look something like this. "Well, I would say *this* to you, to which you would respond to me in *THIS* way. The whole issue would be recognized and dismissed, so why bother saying anything when it will all just blow over anyhow." Oh-oh.... We all know what suppression can lead to. MOUNT VESUVIUS!!

8

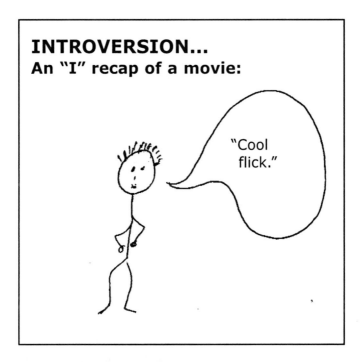

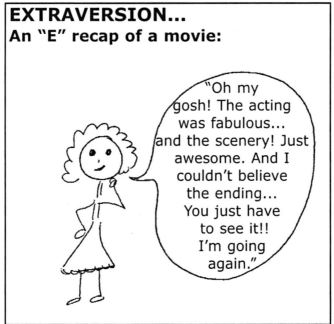

CONVERSATION ETIQUETTE

When two Extraverts are conversing, there can be a lot of talking over one another. They may be so excited about what THEY want to contribute that they don't hear a word the other person is saying. Attention needs to be given not only to allowing the other party to speak, but to actually LISTENING to what is being said. A good way to remind yourself of this if you happen to be an animated Extravert is to stop talking and breathe. Not only will the communication be much more meaningful, you will be doing something healthy for yourself at the same time. Similar steps should be taken when an Extravert and Introvert exchange information as well, because as you can imagine, the Introvert might not even get a chance to say "boo."

Now when two Introverts are 'conversing' there is the possibility, unless they are both mind readers, that some pertinent information could be missed. If something of real importance is to be shared, they might actually consider communicating in writing. This will give both parties the opportunity to ponder what it is being relayed as well as time to respond honestly.

This reminds me of a time when "Instant Messaging" had just come into being and I happened to be online at the same time as my very dear friend, Beth, who was living in Taiwan. We hadn't corresponded in quite a while and when we recognized we were both 'available for contact,' it was indeed INSTANT 'communication'... Both being Es, we proceeded to ask questions, answer questions and literally 'write' all over each other!! Anyone else trying to follow the story line would probably have become dizzy, but we were just communicating the way two Extraverts do, especially when they haven't seen one another in a while!

MEETING TIP

If you wish to get the most out of your meetings, be they your once-a-week family/tribal gatherings or your employee conferences, you will do everyone a favor if you publish your agenda in advance. This will prove effective in not only streamlining the tete-a-tete but will also give any Introverts attending a much firmer foundation from which to share. Without this 'preview' you will most likely have the Extraverts talking over one another while the Is sit with crossed arms wishing they were on a desert island or anywhere else for that matter, as long as it is far away from there. You may also miss out on some potentially important information if you are gathering data from only one side of the group.

IN A NUTSHELL...

EXTRAVERTS
* Are energized by the outer world of people and things
* Have a vocal thought process
* Make experiences 'real' by sharing them
* Sometimes think out loud to the confusion of those around them

INTROVERTS
* Are energized by the inner world and quiet time
* Have an internal thought process
* Don't need to share an experience to make it 'real'
* Sometimes hold important information inside them creating confusion

---

SENSORS (S) & INTUITIVES (N)*
- How We Perceive Reality
* We use 'N' to indicate iNtuitive because the I is associated with Introversion.

This preference is typically the starting point where communication can go awry. If you and I are looking at the same thing and seeing something different, that would be the first clue. A very major point needs to be made here. This does not mean that one person is right and the other wrong. It just means we see things in different ways. This understanding can be invaluable in keeping lines of communication open.

Reality for the Sensor is typically based on what they perceive through their **five senses.** What they can see, hear, touch, taste and smell is REAL for them. Because of this, they also tend to trust past experience over a 'gut feeling' because it is something that has proven itself to be true (at least then) vs the parameters of the 'unknown.'

The iNtuitive, on the other hand, also takes information in through the five senses, but they then relate this to a **bigger picture.** An N can walk right by something without seeing it if they are somewhere else in their mind. One of my 'iNuitive experiences' comes to mind here as an example. One evening while living in Germany, a group of us had gone bowling. Being an amateur as well as a bit of a perfectionist (dangerous combination), I was determined to get a strike or at the very least, a few spares. Well, my opportunity presented itself. Nine pins down, one to go... I became SO fixated on the last standing pin that I drew the ball back and just as I was releasing it to capture my moment of glory, my husband screamed "NOOOOOOOOO!!!" It was rather like a slow motion scene from a movie as I realized that the gate in front of the pin had NOT yet gone

12

up and my 14 pound bowling ball was careening down the lane at the speed of a bullet (well, it SEEMED like that) and finally fully engaged the gate. By this time, we had the attention of all the other bowlers who watched in amused anticipation. BOOOOM!!! So much for my athletic performance. My N had betrayed me. HOW could I have not seen that gate? Well, because I had already 'seen' the spare and the little dance I was going to do afterward in celebration. (Quite embarrassing.)

GENERALITIES VS SPECIFICS

There are many levels on which the S and the N can misunderstand one another. One would be the perception of time. The Sensor is much more in tune to the present and not particularly enamored with long range planning. The iNtuitive perceives time in a more random manner. (This perception can also be magnified by another of our preferences, the J/P line, but we will discuss that in just a bit. Oh - "just a bit" - that would be a perfect example of an N's relation to time. "How LONG is 'just a bit'?" most Sensors would inquire. "5 minutes? An hour? A DAY???" They really do like specifics. That's why they should also be the ones to balance the check book. ("What do you MEAN you just round it off?!")

Both of my parents were Sensors and it was quite evident when they would give people directions to their home in California. They lived in a gated community and Dad would tell friends, "When you get to the entryway, we live 1.9 miles from there."

Their iNtuitive daughter would sometimes test the waters to determine who really was paying attention to detail (and this years before becoming involved with this instrument). In my college dorm, I would hang a sign on one of the elevators (of which there were two) that read, " THIS ELEVATOR IS IN ORDER." It was quite comical to watch the number of people who avoided the 'in order' elevator. My guess, mostly iNtuitives. The Sensors actually read the sign. Perplexed, perhaps. But happy the elevator was working.

S-N Scenario... A couple of friends came over for dinner one spring evening and related that earlier that day they had booked a Caribbean cruise for the coming fall. Jenny, who happened to be an N, was looking at a world map I had on the wall and animatedly pointed out to her husband Ray all the islands they would be visiting. Ray, an S, looked at her patronizingly and said, "Sweetheart, we aren't GOING for over 6 months." To which the N replied, "Does that mean I can't start looking forward to it yet?" For the iNtuitive, she was already there. Sunshine, beaches, and pina coladas. For the Sensor, it would become 'reality' when he set foot on the ship.

SENSING...
An "S" gives driving directions:

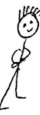 Get in your car. Turn on ignition. Go 3 blocks and turn left at the blue house. Continue on for 1.25 miles and get on interstate going north. Drive 3.75 miles and take the Main Street exit. Go left and follow the road to a T and turn right. Five houses down on your left you will see a yellow home with a rose bushes and a green Chevy parked in the driveway. Stop there.

INTUITION...
An "N" gives driving directions:

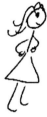

Drive about a 1/2 mile
and get on the interstate
Take the Chicago exit
and go left.
You can't miss it.

Though our differences may be quite apparent, we can indeed learn a lot from one another and also form excellent teams. The Sensor is involved in the moment and the detail, but not thrilled about projecting too far down the line. The iNtuitive likes nothing better than to imagine the future and turn dreams into reality. Working and living together can assist both types in 'seeing' beyond their comfort zones and achieving goals.

IN A NUTSHELL...

SENSORS
* Take information in through their 5 senses
* Prefer to trust past experience over 'gut' feelings
* Have a tendency to take things literally
* Work well with detail

INTUITIVES
* Take information in through their 5 senses and relate it to a bigger picture
* Tend to live in the future
* Look at the world of possibilities
* Trust their hunches

THINKERS (T) & FEELERS (F)
- How We Make Our Decisions

Once again, a prologue prior to further discussion... The terms for this preference are based on Jungian theory and were the words that Jung himself chose to represent the process. Considering the connotations of each of these in 'regular' usage, they may conjure up a quite inaccurate supposition. The point I would like to make here is that Thinkers do indeed have feelings and Feelers also use an objective, logical thought process. There. Now we can proceed.

This preference has everything to do with our comfort zone regarding decision-making. They are both rational foundations from which to base our decisions and we all do both, BUT one will almost always be more comfortable than the other. We can even come to like conclusions as Ts and Fs, but we will have very different ways of getting there. For instance, in her book entitled *You Just Don't Understand*, Dr. Deborah Tannen, tells the story of a radio talk show host interviewing the parents of an autistic child. She asks them if there is ever a time when they start feeling sorry for themselves because of the life situation they are experiencing. The mother, who happened to be a Feeler, answered "No." She explained that the one she felt empathy for was her son because he was the one who was enduring the frustration and pain on a daily basis. When the father, who happened to be a Thinker, answered the question, he also said "No." But *his* explanation was that "life is full of problems and this was just one more problem to solve."[1] So, while they were in agreement that they did not feel sorry for themselves, their reasoning for reaching that conclusion was poles apart.

16

BASIC DIFFERENCES... OBJECTIVITY VS SUBJECTIVITY

Thinkers are usually quite capable of separating themselves from an issue and in that distance come to resolution. They may appear cool or aloof in the process, but this does not mean that they are cold-hearted (or possibly in the eyes of the Feeler, "Out to get me!") They just feel more 'at home' with a logical, objective stance and are often confused about why the Feeler always takes everything so personally.

When Feelers come to decisions, they most often find themselves becoming a part of the situation. It is more difficult for them to distance themselves from what is happening as they take a more subjective viewpoint. They may appear wishy-washy to those observing their process, but once again, this would be an uninformed assumption. For the Feeler, this is also where the 'objective' practice of constructive criticism becomes an oxymoron. If you criticize a Feeler, you can almost always expect hurt feelings.

This is indeed why learning about type is so very eye-opening. Knowing how another processes information and comes to a decision can greatly reduce the time one spends in the land of 'blame.'

> Of note...Statistics have shown that our population is divided roughly 50-50 in terms of percentages regarding the Thinking / Feeling preference but of interest is that approximately 2/3 of Thinkers are male and 2/3 of Feelers are female.

When I married the first time... (Okay. Wait. It's time to divulge more personal stuff.) I have borrowed a wonderful line from a dear friend when I explain that I have 'successfully completed two marriages.' All the more ammunition for teaching about type, right?) ANYHOW... Where was I? Oh yeah. The first marriage: As a Feeler, I entered the realm of Thinkers. My husband and his entire family were all Ts. I could almost hear the unspoken question that was running through each of their logical heads, "WHO IS THIS PERSON THAT WANTS TO KEEP HUGGING US?" While it was obvious that a lot of love was felt between them, it was not something that was vocalized or overtly shown, where in my own household, you didn't even THINK of going to bed without a good night kiss and an "I love you." (If company was visiting, they all got a kiss, too.)

I had lot to learn about Ts. And a lot to learn FROM them as well. Because, as with all of the preferences, our type opposites can be wonderful teachers. If we are to achieve balance or 'Individuation' as Carl Jung referred to this concept, we need to learn to be conversant in both our preferred modes of action as well as the contrasting.

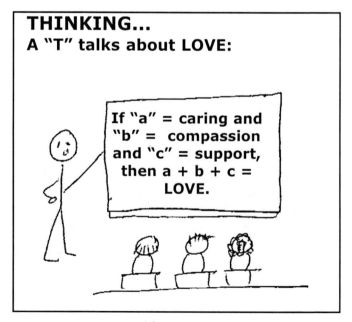

THINKING...
A "T" talks about LOVE:

If "a" = caring and "b" = compassion and "c" = support, then a + b + c = LOVE.

FEELING...
An "F" talks about LOVE:

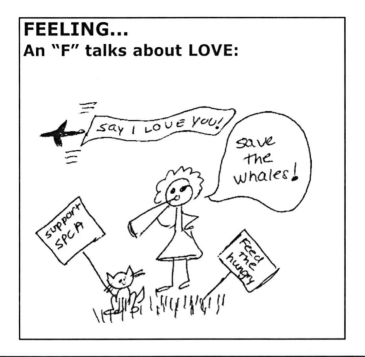

IN THE WORKPLACE

A scenario that might appear familiar unfolds in a workplace where a Feeling employee named Lucy is diligently attending to paperwork at her desk. Martha, her Thinking boss walks in, goes right past the F without saying good morning and closes her office door. This is not 'normal' behavior for the boss as every other morning she has greeted Lucy with a smile and asked how she is doing. Right away, Lucy is sure that she has done something to precipitate this change in conduct. Her mind and heart race to identify what she could have done to get on her boss's bad side. Did she forget a work assignment? Handle a phone call in too abrupt a manner? Maybe she isn't dressed properly for the job!! All of these scripts ricochet off the walls of Lucy's brain like a pinball machine out of control... when all along it could very well be that Martha just has a whole lot on her mind. Oh, the anguish we can avoid when we practice open communication...

The preceding story suggests invaluable information when dealing not only with employees and colleagues, but also with friends and family. Before jumping to conclusions, it is always best to be honest and open in the lines of communication, especially when behavior is uncharacteristic. Again, one of the primary benefits of becoming familiar with how opposite types operate is that their behavior tends to make a lot more sense *and* we can also learn to use the terminology that taps into that wavelength (the radio frequency).

IN A NUTSHELL...

THINKERS
* Make decisions from an objective viewpoint
* Prefer logic over feeling
* Could come across as cold or aloof

FEELERS
* Make decisions from a subjective viewpoint
* Prefer feeling over logic
* Could come across as wishy-washy

JUDGERS (J) & PERCEIVERS (P)
- Lifestyle Choices: So, How Do YOU Feel About Lists?

This particular preference may be one of the easiest to spot whether you are dealing with friends, family and co-workers or even with complete strangers. Js or Judgers have a distinct partiality for 'wrapping things up.' Open ends make them uncomfortable. Because of this, they can seem overly anal at times in their desire for closure.

As an example, when my husband and I were making a move from Norfolk, Virginia to Washington, D.C. where neither of us had lived before, I was quite anxious about getting things firmed up as far as housing was concerned. It was February and we were due to move in July. We were made aware of a house that was for rent (we weren't planning on staying so buying was not an option) and I suggested we make the 3 hour drive to investigate. It turned out to be a very nice home in a pretty neighborhood, had a great yard for Chica, our golden retriever (high priority) and was also not too far from the Pentagon where he would be working. Overall, a complete match. So, I announced in my Extraverted-Judger way, "This is it. Let's sign." To which my Perceiver husband replied, "How can we possibly sign? This is the first one we have looked at and we have nothing to compare it to!!"

This should give you a hint to the modus operandi of the P or Perceiving Type. Closure is what you come to when ALL options have been exhausted. They are very big on putting things down in pencil (if at all) in case 'something better comes up.' Commitment is something you do when there are no alternatives left to explore.

TRAVELING Js

After going through a divorce (and no, it had nothing to do with the house in D.C.) I was dating a guy from New York. My parents were still not very happy about the split up and had yet to meet my boyfriend. They were coming to my home in Nashville to visit and he was feeling quite nervous about their first meeting. To make matters worse, the plane was delayed which led to excessive pacing and sighing as we awaited their arrival. (This was back in the 'good ol' days' when you could actually meet someone at their gate.) Well, finally the plane landed, Mom and Dad disembarked and after the preliminary hugs, we all walked toward baggage claim, Mom and I, of course, talking up a storm. Dad announced that he was going to get the rental car and would meet us at the carousel. When we got there my boyfriend offered to get the bags off the conveyor and Mom said, "Oh, they should be very easy to recognize. They each have a big red ribbon tied to the handle." As we continued our conversation, he watched for the luggage. Here comes one with a red ribbon... takes it off. Here comes another with a red ribbon, takes it off. Here comes ANOTHER... AND ANOTHER...all bearing red ribbons!! At this point, he is thinking, "My God!! How long are they staying?!!!" Just about then Mom glanced up and said, "Those aren't our bags!!" Well, apparently there had been an article the weekend prior in the Sunday Parade section of the newspaper sharing a 'handy little hint' for making your luggage easy to identify. (AND apparently Mom and Dad were not the only Js to read the article.) Quite humorous.

WHAT'S ON *YOUR* CALENDAR?

Ps can actually feel quite impressed with themselves believing that they are accomplishing a lot as they begin one project and then another and then another... but key here is, are ANY of them getting completed? The J can feel quite proud that they have COMPLETED a project in record time, but if they have cut corners or ignored possible repercussions, their handiwork may just have to be repeated. So much for time management. Taking this into consideration, how can we learn from one another? The P can prevent the J from closing prematurely and the J can bring the meandering P to conclusions.

Both of my parents were 'off-the-wall' Js and one of the J's FAVORITE things to do in life is to make a list and THEN cross off whatever they have accomplished. (Dad would actually make lists for the entire family. Not everyone was as thrilled.) Many Js may even go so far as to ADD things to the list that they have done along the way so that they can cross those off as well... And yes, as a J myself, I'm guilty as charged. It just produces *such* a feeling of satisfaction. (REARRANGED CAT FOOD CANS IN CUPBOARD - CHECK!!)

The Perceiver for the most part finds the whole list thing either tedious, a distraction or just a waste of time. How can you 'go with the flow' if you have to follow a schedule? Once again you can see the lessons we can learn. Schedules are crucial to most of our lives if we are to navigate through our days in a smooth manner. But like anything else, planning can be overdone leading to zero spontaneity. (And by the way, Js, it doesn't count if you write *this* on your to-do list: "Tomorrow at 2:15 p.m., I will be spontaneous.")

Going with the flow is not only creatively inspiring, it is also healthy. "Embracing the moment..." But again, without some parameters and setting of goals, life can pass you by and leave you looking at a lot of missed opportunities. Balance, sweet balance.

JUDGING ...
A "J" shares their Saturday to do list:

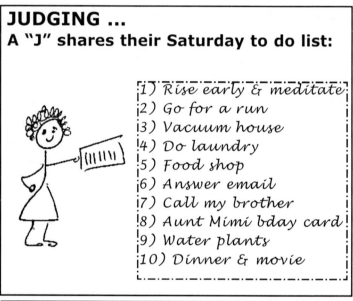

1) Rise early & meditate
2) Go for a run
3) Vacuum house
4) Do laundry
5) Food shop
6) Answer email
7) Call my brother
8) Aunt Mimi bday card
9) Water plants
10) Dinner & movie

PERCEIVING ...
A "P" shares their Saturday to do list:

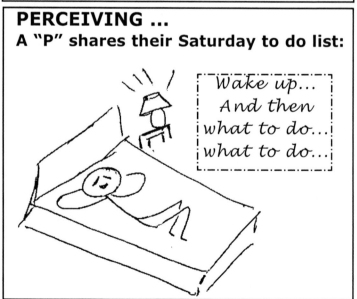

Wake up...
And then
what to do...
what to do...

IN A NUTSHELL...

JUDGERS
* Love structure and calendars
* Know that a to-do list is the only way to stay organized
* May come to closure too soon in the interest of 'wrapping things up.'

PERCEIVERS
* Are flexible and spontaneous
* May be easily distracted and/or absent-minded
* Prefer to explore all options before coming to closure

INDIVIDUATION... Getting to know 'YOU'

Balance in all preferences is key to personal growth. We all have our comfort zones, to be sure, but getting to know the opposite preference can be helpful in many ways. Not only do we become more adept at weighing the pros and cons of a situation, we will also find it easier to understand and communicate with others in our lives who embrace preferences different from our own.

The expression "Individuation" itself is a Jungian term. Of utmost importance in our life journey, is the discovery and realization of SELF, the moment-by-moment adventure in the unfolding of our soul's potential. Beautifully stated by Sue Monk Kidd in her book, *When the Heart Waits*, she writes, "You've probably noticed how window plants wind and grow toward the light, pressing leaves against the pane. This turning toward the sun has a scientific name; it's called *heliotropism*. Jung spoke of a 'human heliotropism.' The True Self seeks the light, winding and growing toward realization, pressing against the window pane of consciousness."[2] How utterly beautifully stated.

By getting to know ourselves from the inside out, we not only build our awareness of opposites, thereby increasing empathy, but also heighten our own ability to endure the inevitable twists and turns of life.

In workshops we often do an exercise where we first write our names with our preferred hand. It's easy; no need to give it any thought. We then switch to our less-preferred hand and again sign our name. When asked for a description of how this feels, the usual responses are "awkward, strange, uncomfortable, impossible" and so on. The analogy is clear. One must first be AWARE of the 'other side of the coin' and then it requires practice and patience to become adept at making the most of this knowledge or activity.

> "I use the term 'individuation' to denote the process by which a person becomes a psychological 'in-divid-ual,' that is, a separate, indivisible unity or 'whole.'"
> - C. G. Jung[3]

Team Captain, Co-captain (and oh, yeah.. that Benchwarmer guy)

No matter your type, we each have what are referred to as DOMI-NANT, AUXILIARY, TERTIARY AND INFERIOR FUNC-TIONS. These functions relate to the middle two letters of our type and represent the 'batting order' or partiality regarding the sequence in their usage. Let me first give you a broad overview and then we will get into specifics.

Our dominant function, or the "team captain" so to speak, will be the process that you rely on most heavily. Depending on whether you are an Extravert or an Introvert this preference of choice will either be outwardly expressed for the world to see (E) or internally experienced where it is kept under wraps (I).

Our auxiliary function, the "co-captain," is the next in the pecking order of reliance. It is exactly the opposite as far as what the world sees, for example, the auxiliary function for the Extravert will be an internal process and for the Introvert this preference will be more openly demonstrated.

Our tertiary function will be third in line when being looked to for guidance. And finally, our inferior function being last on the list, is usually tackled somewhat later in life but could also be ignored all together, ergo, the "benchwarmer" status. Let's take a look at a specific four-letter type, for example an ESTJ, to get an idea of this pecking order. (We will be reviewing all 16 types later in the book.)

ESTJ: Extraverted - Sensing - Thinking - Judger

As an Extravert, the team captain - or dominant function - will be the THINKING preference (T). The world will be exposed to your decision-making process and will probably hear structure and a need for closure. Second in line, your auxiliary or co-captain will be your SENSING preference (S). This will be an internal process, so as you form your decisions outwardly, you will attend to the details within. The third function you access will be your INTUITION (N) - (the opposite of your auxiliary) which, as an Extravert will again be shown to the world. In this case, one will most likely hear you speaking of possibilities, future references and so on... although THIS IS NOT your preference (Sensing is.) And finally, on to your inferior function of Feeling (F) which will revert back to an internal process. Interpersonal issues may take a back seat to rules and regulations.

There are many resources for delving more deeply into the mechanics behind this theory and I will therefore not be going into further explanation here. I do, though, find it relevant to share the general guidelines because it does indeed explain why certain types may 'appear' different than what one would expect when their type is known.

TYPE AND AGE

Of particular interest is that as we age, each of our functions becomes more highly activated. Because I believe we are actually born with our Type already determined, the basic blueprint has thus been drawn up, so to speak. But as a general guideline, we also tend to develop each of these functions during different time periods in life.

The dominant function, quite naturally, will be the first to develop and usually becomes more apparent from the age of ten through twenty years. The auxiliary function will begin to ask for more attention between the ages of twenty and thirty. The tertiary function may start becoming more pronounced between the ages of thirty and forty and finally, the inferior function, again, last to 'join the party' may finally kick in sometime around midlife. This is a very general timeline, as events and circumstances may have effects that can either emphasize the evolution or stifle the development of the various functions at different times along our life course.

What I find important to recognize is that though our dominant will always be the most comfortable and preferred of the functions, it could appear to take a leave of absence as the others vie for attention. This could result in what appears to be some very uncharacteristic behavior. So, it's nice to have a possible explanation for why Aunt Jessie is wearing miniskirts to church on Sunday.

LITTLE (FUN) DISCLAIMER FROM AUTHOR

For those NTs (iNtuitive Thinkers) with perfectionist tendencies as well as any detail-oriented Ss (Sensors) AND/OR structure-loving Js (Judgers), if you happen to find a typo here or there within these pages, please just deal with it. I've done my best to produce an 'error free' manuscript and, indeed, being a sensitive F (Feeler), you know how we react to criticism.

ON TO THE CHAKRAS...

Now that we have a bit of background regarding the 'building blocks' of Type, let's proceed to an introduction to our energy fields before reviewing the individual profiles. This knowledge will tie into the balancing gifts that the chakra toolkits will have to offer for each of the sixteen types.

CHAPTER 2

Our Chakras:
The Building Blocks of Our Energy Sytem

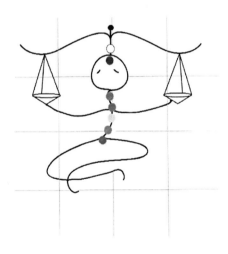

Let your energy
flow with the wind,
And your path will find YOU,
again and again.
                    - Maureen

Introducing... Our Beautiful Chakras

Now we will enter the world of energy and begin to explore how our innate personalities can affect the flow of that life force within us.

The word "chakra" is Sanskrit for wheel or disc and refers to the seven main fields of energy located in our etheric (subtle) body, the reservoir of our life force. These spinning vortices form the doorway between the mind and the body and are focal points for the reception and transmission of this energy. The etheric body itself is the same shape as our physical body and extends out from this form housing these wheels that are situated along the spinal column.

If we are well-balanced, "prana" or life force energy flows unimpeded along its course within us, resulting in health from physical and emotional perspectives. The psychologist C. G. Jung called the chakras the "portals to consciousness," and saw each of these fields as "universes unto themselves" that reflected the process of individuation, the development of the individual personality.

The most comprehensive and clear explanations of the chakra system that I have found belong to Anodea Judith. As Judith states in her book *Chakra Balancing*, "Just as the electricity running through your computer allows your software and your hardware to work together effectively, the mind (software) and the body (hardware) are brought together by the life force running through you." [1]

I think it is sometimes difficult for us to wrap our minds around this whole concept and what has made it more accessible to me is the following theory from Dr. David R. Hamilton in his ground-breaking book, *How Your Mind Can Heal Your Body*: "If you look inside your body, you see cells. If you look inside cells, you find molecules, of which DNA is one. Looking at what DNA is made of, you learn that it's atoms. But if you look inside the atom, it's mostly empty space... Subatomic particles (protons, neutrons, electons and so on) are not particles at all. You see, they aren't solid but are actually vibrations of energy... The bottom line is that reality is not solid, but is constructed from vibrations of energy."[2]

The FACT that we are made up of energy makes the connection to our chakra system a much more comfortable leap. Energetic fields within our body control, enable and prosper our health and well-being in a variety of ways.

LET IT FLOW!

All of the chakras are interrelated and when an imbalance occurs in one, it will have residual effects all along the energy pathway. These imbalances can occur when energy flows either too strongly *or* too weakly and sometimes a channel can be blocked entirely. A great analogy shared by various teachers, is that of a garden hose that has been sitting outside all winter. The first time you try to water your spring flowers, the flow from the spigot will most likely cough and sputter as it tries to maneuver its way past the mud, leaves and guck that have accumulated all winter long. Once the hose is cleared, however, the water flows freely. This is our goal as well. Remove the 'guck' and let it flow!

My goal is to introduce you to specific areas in our bodies that can become 'clogged' like that garden hose and how our personalities can influence where these blockages are most likely to occur. The recognition of your innate STRENGTHS is also of huge relevance, as you come to realize how maintenance of certain chakras will keep you tuned in to attributes that can greatly enhance your personal life path.

A BRIEF RECAP OF THE SEVEN MAIN FIELDS

We will be going into much more depth later in the book regarding each of the chakras, but I would like to provide you here with a snapshot view of the seven main fields.

1) **ROOT CHAKRA:** Our first chakra is located at the base of the spine and is the seat of stability and grounding.

2) **SACRAL CHAKRA:** Our second chakra is located in the sacral/pelvic region of our body and is the seat of creation and flow.

3) **SOLAR PLEXUS CHAKRA:** Our third chakra is located in the solar plexus region of the body (behind stomach and just below diaphragm) and is the seat of inner power and self-esteem.

4) **HEART CHAKRA:** Our fourth chakra is located in the heart/chest area and is the seat of love and compassion.

5) THROAT CHAKRA: Our fifth chakra is located in the throat region, also housing the thyroid gland, shoulder and neck region and is the seat of communication and self-expression.

6) THIRD EYE CHAKRA: Our sixth chakra is located between the brows and is the seat of intuition.

7) CROWN CHAKRA: Our seventh chakra is located at the top of the head and is the seat of our connection to the Divine.

TOOLKITS

Following the overview of the sixteen personality profiles, I will acquaint you with 'toolkits' for each of the chakras. The kits will include specific yoga postures, breathing practices (pranayama) meditations, affirmations, and mudras (seals or 'hand yoga' - see below for further explanation) and will complement each particular field. These will be divided into three realms:

1) Inborn areas of strength that can be maintained through this chakra's toolkit
2) Areas that are in a weakened state and in need of additional energy
3) Areas where the energy in a particular field may be flowing too strongly and you will be referred to a different toolkit to reestabish harmony

MUDRAS

According to Gertrud Hirschi, author of Mudras - Yoga in Your Hands, "... mudras engage certain areas of the brain and/or soul and exercise a corresponding influence on them. However, mudras are also effective on the phsysical level... We can often engage and influence our body and our mind by bending, crossing, extending or touching the fingers with other fingers."[3]

So, how long should a mudra be held?

Again, according to Hirschi, if you are experiencing a 'chronic' symptom, you can hold the position up to 45 minutes (or 3 x 15 minutes) per day. For more 'acute' complaints, holding between 3 and 30 minutes should be sufficient. I personally believe holding them for even a minute - or less than that during the yoga flow - as long as it is done in conjunction with breath and intention, will bring about results, possibly subtle at first but eliciting positive repercussions nonetheless.

And now, let's move on to the profiles!

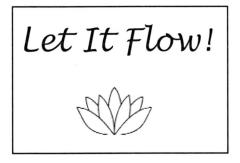

Find that place between
'trying and not' -
where dreams become real
and the dance is taught.
                    - Maureen

CHAPTER 3

Overview of the Sixteen Personality Profiles

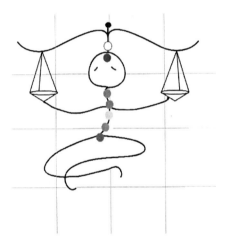

We will now take a look at each of the sixteen different Personality Types and the relevant Chakra Balancing Toolkits that will help celebrate, maintain and restore balance. The following section of the book will then introduce you to the toolkits themselves.

ENERGY TYPES

ISTJ (Introverted-Sensing-Thinking-Judger) - Just Don't Surprise Me

Welcome to the world of what could be the most private of all of the types. As a dominant (introverted) Sensor, the universe of detail that surrounds us at any given moment will be their first stopping off point. They take in bits and pieces of information that other types might not see even if held point blank in front of them! This gathering of facts, figures and miscellaneous particulars will then be processed and filed into the databank of knowledge within the brain of the ISTJ. Should they need to access any piece of this cataloged data, it will be generated with nary a thought. Order and precision are of extreme importance to this type.

If you live with an ISTJ, you are probably familiar with their attachment to lists and agendas. Punctuality is not just something that you practice to be polite, but rather an expected behavior on all accounts. And we are not just talking roundabout... we are talking down to minutes and seconds. If you plan to leave the house at 8:32 a.m., then that is when you will leave. NOT 8:29 a.m. and NOT 8:35 a.m. Get it?

The ISTJ will not usually find themselves wasting any energy on looking for something they have lost or misplaced because they know that things are to be put away where they belong once you are through using them. Oh, and speaking of 'things'... If you have 'things' that haven't been used in 10 months, 3 weeks and 5 days, you will most likely not need them at any time in the future either. So, you might as well throw out, recycle or gift them to someone who may find a use for them. (If you are a closet hoarder, better make sure it's a space the ISTJ does not have access to.)

These characteristics also make the ISTJ one of the most responsible of the types. If they say they are going to be somewhere or if they offer assitance with a project or function, they will be there on time and ready to support the cause.

Under stress, the ISTJ may initially become even more introverted and structured. If the stress continues to escalate, however, you may see a metamorphosis that causes them to throw caution to the wind. Lists be banished! The time is now! (Quite contrary to their natural desire for control and for that reason a bit scary as well.)

Regarding control, the ISTJ is not one who typically finds surprises to be a fun thing. If you are going to spring something unplanned on this type, you had better tell them about it beforehand. (I know, then it's not really a surprise. But believe me, it's just easier this way.)

In intimate relationships, it may take the ISTJ a bit of time before feeling comfortable enough to share information regarding their personal life. Even years. When they do make a commitment, however, it is written in stone. While romance might not be tops on their agenda, you can usually expect a faithful, devoted partner at your side. As is the case with most S-Js (Sensing-Judgers), tradition is quite important to them and this will be readily apparent in the upbringing of their children as well. This is the way I did it as a kid, so why change anything if it worked for me?

Careerwise, the ISTJ would be most validated in an environment that is structured and stable. Accounting, military, clerical/administrative work, and management are areas that might fit the bill.

Private, detail-oriented and dependable, the ISTJ adds organization and calm to an often less-than predictable world.

HIERARCHY OF FUNCTION ("Who's On First?")

The middle two letters of a person's type - our 'functions' - will equate to how we experience (perceive) reality and how we make our decisions. The 'authority' as to which of these processes occurs first will vary by type. There is an order we go through when accessing them and this is pretty much determined by the 'comfort zones' of our individual type.

We each have...
a DOMINANT FUNCTION (Team Captain)
an AUXILIARY FUNCTION (Co-captain)
a TERTIARY FUNCTION (Third at bat)
and an INFERIOR FUNCTION (Benchwarmer)

Of note, the Extravert (E) will 'share' their dominant process with the world and internalize their auxiliary. The Introvert (I) will do the opposite, keeping their most preferred function internal and showing the world the 'next in command.'

This is the breakdown fo the ISTJ:
DOMINANT (introverted) S
AUXILIARY (extraverted) T
TERTIARY (introverted) F
INFERIOR (introverted) N

Type Preference by Letter for the ISTJ:

E/I (Extraversion /Introversion): *How we are energized...* If you choose **Introversion** over Extraversion, you are usually most energized when spending quiet time alone or in the company of one or two close friends. You process things internally which Extraverts often find frustrating as they are not being kept up to date with minute by minute proceedings. If you want the most truthful, complete answer from an I, give them time to withdraw from the ruckus of the outer world and go within. Introverts also do not have the need to share their entire life story with people in line at the bank or sitting next to them on a plane. They are usually quite content to exist in their own universe until a need is felt to 'come out and play.' Now Introverts also need people, but being around too many people for too long a time can physically make them wither. As with any of the preferences, preservation of health means maintaining balance.

S/N (Sensing/iNtuition): *How we perceive reality...* This preference boils down to how we take in information, a vital component in communication. If we are experiencing *different* realities, learning to see things through the eyes of the receiving party will enable us to share in a way that will be understood. If you choose **Sensing** over iNtuition, you are probably very engaged in the world of detail, the past and day-to-day experience. Living in the present and in the tactile world of the five senses - i.e. what you see, hear, taste, smell and touch - is your reality and you are quite attuned to your environment. (This in comparison to the iNtuitive who resides in the realm of possibilities, trusts 'gut feelings' over past experience, is future-oriented and not always cognizant of what is going on in the physical world. They tend to live beyond the 5 senses.) Being practical and dealing

with 'what is' as opposed to 'what could be' are key attributes of the Sensing Type. The S may also take things quite literally which the N should keep in mind when sharing information as miscommunication *could* run rampant. ("You SAID be here on the hour... but you DIDN'T say which one!") All in all, they can make great partners, but understanding the different modes of perception is essential.

T/F (Thinking/Feeling): *How we make our decisions...* These are both rational means of decision-making but one will almost always offer a much more natural approach. When **Thinking** is preferred over Feeling (again please recall that these are Jungian terms and don't indicate that we don't all do both) the decisions will be more from the head than the heart as the T tends to take an objective stance apart from the situation vs becoming embedded in the process. While we all practice both modes of determination and one will be more natural, it is highly beneficial to learn to look at both sides of an issue, subjectively as well as objectively. In the world of the Feeler, this is where things like "constructive criticism" become an oxymoron. If you are critical of an F from any standpoint, you can almost be certain they will be hurt. One of the biggest gifts the MBTI® offers, is the understanding of *why* we process certain things the way we do. Subsequently, in this situation, the Feeler could learn that yes, it is okay to decide with your heart, but don't forget to balance it out by taking a step back and viewing the situation from the perspective of an observer. This is also helpful when dealing with Thinkers who may appear harsh or overly critical. Once it's understood that this is a decision making PROCESS, and not meant to be accusatory, these two preference types can come to much better understanding. (The same being true for the Thinker dealing with the Feeler: "Why do you take everything to heart?") In truth, as in all preference pairings, we can learn so much from one another.

J/P (Judging/Perceiving): *Our lifestyle...* Choosing **Judging** over Perceiving usually indicates a preference for closure, structure and lists. "Let's wrap it up" could be the motto of most Js. Open ends tend to make them uncomfortable. Now many times, especially for the Feeling-Judger, this could mean coming to closure just to avoid hurt feelings or any kind of conflict. (Which, depending on the situation, means you may end up having to deal with the scenario all over again.) This is in contrast to the P who prefers flexibility and leaving the door open until all options have been studied (or playing what I refer to as "ostrich." This entails putting your head in the ground and avoiding the fact that a decision even needs to be made.) Judgers like to live by a list and get a sense of achievement with crossing something off of that list. When living with a P, they may become critical if things aren't returned to their original place and also wonder why the P can't make simple decisions. (And the J knows exactly which way the TP and paper towels should come over the roll.) All in all, the J can lend structure and stability to just about any situation, and this is a wonderful trait, as long as they remain open to allowing for inevitable change.

ISTJ, CHAKRAS & BALANCE

I will now acquaint you with suggested toolkits for the **ISTJ** that will include specific yoga postures, breathing practices (Pranayama) meditations, affirmations, and mudras (seals or 'hand yoga').

After an explanation of the 'toolkits' I have chosen to help enhance and maintain your natural strength as well as regain balance when necessary, there will be a short series of questions you can ask yourself to clarify just which energy field is most in need of attention.

Suggested Toolkits to Celebrate, Nurture & Restore Balance:
Root Chakra, Sacral Chakra Third Eye Chakra
(Depending on your particular life situation, ANY of the chakras may 'deserve' attention. You can determine this by reviewing the questions found in each toolkit.)

As a dominant Sensor (S) combined with co-captain Thinking (T) AND Judging (J) preference, your strengths are found in your stability and groundedness. Working with the **ROOT CHAKRA TOOLKIT** will support those innate gifts and allow you to make make the most of them. This is also a flow you can turn to if you are feeling LESS than grounded, in order to reestablish that footing.

The combination of Sensing-Judging (S-J) could also precipitate a need for spending time in the **SACRAL CHAKRA TOOLKIT** to provide you with a sense of movement and flow. While stability can be a very positive thing, if the roots become so entrenched that you feel 'pot-bound' your ability to deal with change could be greatly impaired. You may also find yourself stuck in the doldrums and unable to access your sense of motivation. This flow can greatly enhance those areas of your life.

While your natural inclinations will celebrate your ability to provide support and foundations within your life, you may also find spending time in the **THIRD EYE CHAKRA TOOLKIT** to be beneficial. Embrace this internal realm, especially if you are in the middle of any situation that demands relying on your intuition. 'Ajna' will make sure that you are seeing the whole picture and taking various possibilities into account. This will prevent coming to closure too soon which can quickly turn a decision into a 'whoops' moment.

47

All types need to be cognizant of the role that the throat chakra plays in our ability to communicate. The I-T will need to be wary of avoiding issues because they feel 'uncomfortable' or 'none of my business.' But if areas of discomfort become suppressed rather than expressed, you may find that your health and emotional stability suffer as a result of not speaking your truth.

Questions for the ISTJ to ask themselves to determine which Chakra to nurture:

1) "Am I feeling grounded and able to support the current situations in my life?"

If YES, practice ROOT CHAKRA flows and meditations with the intention of connecting to earth energy and your ability to provide foundation. If NO, practice ROOT CHAKRA toolkit offerings to help bring you back into your natural gifts of stability.

2) "Do I sense a need to explore beyond the daily list of to-dos and access a deeper sense of inner vision?"

If YES, practice THIRD EYE CHAKRA flows and meditations to embrace the innate sense of intuition that is available to us all when we bring our focus inward. Turn off the static of the outside world as you affirm the guidance that will come when you access this place of knowing.

3) "Am I fearful of change and lacking motivation to move forward in my life?"

If YES, practice SACRAL CHAKRA flows and meditations to bring motion and energy into your being. Keep your own desires and dreams in mind as you allow the motion to set you free.

As always, no matter which energy field we are currently engaging, it is important to hold your intention in both mind and heart and then be open to the inspiration that follows.

ENERGY TYPES

ISFJ (Introverted-Sensing-Feeling-Judger)
- Lovingly Realistic, Realistically Loving

$\mathcal{P}$ractical, realistic, and finding comfort in 'the known and understood,' the ISFJ holds their cards close to the heart. They are able to take in an enormous amount of detail in any given situation and it will be recorded and filed in the library of their psyche where it can be accessed at any given time. Their realism is in constant communion with their feeling nature, and most decisions will revolve around these two arenas: first taking in the data and then subjectively coming to a conclusion.

When life is balanced and they are feeling centered, this can proceed like clockwork. But as we all know, life is subject to change, and change is not high on the list of ISFJ priorities. They in actuality may expend a fair amount of energy attempting to ground both people and situations in their environment which can lead ultimately to exhaustion as they do on some level understand that this endeavor is an impossibility. A suggestion would be to remember that the only 'being' they truly have over control lies within and even in this instance, change is inevitable. Coming to grips with this particular reality can assist them in overcoming that gnawing feeling that the rug is being pulled out from underneath them at random and recurring times.

In social situations, they will most likely sit back and observe, taking everything (and I mean EVERYTHING) in and unless fully at ease in their surroundings will probably just tuck it away for later. If, though, they find themselves in a very 'safe' environment, they may joyfully take advantage of sharing some inner most thoughts and beliefs, but truly only once they are certain that the secrecy is reliable. Because of this, you can count them among your most reliable, trustworthy friends as they will offer you that same confidentiality.

At work, they are a whiz with numbers and detail. They may not have a lot of patience for coworkers who don't appreciate this love of precision and efficiency. In most cases, they are most comfortable in positions that have well-defined expectations as they aren't really fond of being told to 'think outside the box.'

At home, this orderliness is also quite important to them. 'A place for everything and everything in it's place' could definitely be one of their mottos. Because of this desire for structure, tradition within the family unit is of value to them as well.

They can then focus their energy on other areas of strength such as organizing, sharing their calming nature with other less grounded folks and enjoying the earth beneath their feet.

The ISFJ is subject to making mountains out of molehills when there is a communication mix-up. Their Feeling nature, which leads to a propensity for taking things personally, could indeed pick up on a scenario, misread it, and then allow it to fester until it has been blown completely out of proportion. Example: In dealing with a friend who has suggested a night out for dinner and a movie the following week, no further info is transmitted and the date passes without contact. The ISFJ could be known to ingest that data and come to the conclusion that this friend has dumped them and on top of that is probably spreading a number of false rumors about them which will undoubtedly end up on Facebook and THEN... You get the picture. As with all types, communication is a two-way street and words must indeed actually be exchanged for the channels to remain clear. (This is a distinctly perilous area when two Introverts are involved with one another.)

Overall, the ISFJ is a remarkably responsible, caring individual who will give of themselves for the betterment of all concerned, be that in the family or the work environment.

HIERARCHY OF FUNCTION ("Who's On First?")

The middle two letters of a person's type - our 'functions' - will equate to how we experience (perceive) reality and how we make our decisions. The 'authority' as to which of these processes occurs first will vary by type. There is an order we go through when accessing them and this is pretty much determined by the 'comfort zones' of our individual type.

We each have...
a DOMINANT FUNCTION (Team Captain)
an AUXILIARY FUNCTION (Co-captain)
a TERTIARY FUNCTION (Third at bat)
and an INFERIOR FUNCTION (Benchwarmer)

Of note, the Extravert (E) will 'share' their dominant process with the world and internalize their auxiliary. The Introvert (I) will do the opposite, keeping their most preferred function internal and showing the world the 'next in command.'

This is the breakdown fo the ISFJ:
DOMINANT (introverted) S
AUXILIARY (extraverted) F
TERTIARY (introverted) T
INFERIOR (extraverted) N

Type Preference by Letter for the ISFJ:

E/I (Extraversion /Introversion): *How we are energized...*If you choose **Introversion** over Extraversion, you are usually most energized when spending quiet time alone or in the company of one or two close friends. You process things internally which Extraverts often find frustrating as they are not being kept up to date with minute by minute proceedings. If you want the most truthful, complete answer from an I, give them time to withdraw from the ruckus of the outer world and go within. Introverts also do not have the need to share their entire life story with people in line at the bank or sitting next to them on a plane. They are usually quite content to exist in their own universe until a need is felt to 'come out and play.' Now Introverts also need people, but being around too many people for too long a time can physically make them wither. As with any of the preferences, preservation of health means maintaining balance.

S/N (Sensing/iNtuition): *How we perceive reality...* This preference boils down to how we take in information, a vital component in communication. If we are experiencing *different* realities, learning to see things through the eyes of the receiving party will enable us to share in a way that will be understood. If you choose **Sensing** over iNtuition, you are probably very engaged in the world of detail, the past and day-to-day experience. Living in the present and in the tactile world of the five senses - i.e. what you see, hear, taste, smell and touch - is your reality and you are quite attuned to your environment. (This in comparison to the iNtuitive who resides in the realm of possibilities, trusts 'gut feelings' over past experience, is future-oriented and not always cognizant of what is going on in the physical world. They tend to live beyond the 5 senses.) Being practical and dealing with 'what is' as opposed to 'what could be' are key attributes of the

Sensing Type. The S may also take things quite literally which the N should keep in mind when sharing information as miscommunication *could* run rampant. ("You SAID be here on the hour... but you DIDN'T say which one!") All in all, they can make great partners, but understanding the different modes of perception is essential.

T/F (Thinking/Feeling): *How we make our decisions...* If you choose **Feeling** over Thinking as your method of decision making, you tend to become embedded in the situation you are currently encountering. While we all practice both modes of determination, this arena will most often be a more comfortable fit for you. And though one will feel more natural, it is highly beneficial to learn to look at both sides of an issue, subjectively as well as objectively. In the world of the Feeler, this is where things like "constructive criticism" become an oxymoron. If you are critical of an F from any standpoint, you can almost be certain they will be hurt. One of the biggest gifts the MBTI® offers, is the understanding of *why* we process certain things the way we do. For example, in this situation, the Feeler could learn that yes, it is okay to decide with your heart, but don't forget to balance it out by taking a step back, removing yourself as if a bystander. Then take another look at the situation from this perspective. This is also helpful when dealing with Thinkers who may appear harsh or overly critical. Once it's understood that this is a decision making PROCESS, and not meant to be accusatory, these two preference types can come to much better understanding. (The same being true for the Thinker dealing with the Feeler: "Why do you take everything to heart?") In truth, as in all preference pairings, we can learn so much from one another.

J/P (Judging/Perceiving): *Our lifestyle...* Choosing **Judging** over Perceiving usually indicates a preference for closure, structure and lists. "Let's wrap it up" could be the motto of most Js. Open ends tend to make them uncomfortable. Now many times, especially for the Feeling-Judger, this could mean coming to closure just to avoid hurt feelings or any kind of conflict. (Which, depending on the situation, means you may end up having to deal with the scenario all over again.) This is in contrast to the P who prefers flexibility and leaving the door open until all options have been studied (or playing what I refer to as "ostrich." This entails putting your head in the ground and avoiding the fact that a decision even needs to be made.) Judgers like to live by a list and get a sense of achievement with crossing something off of that list. When living with a P, they may become critical if things aren't returned to their original place and also wonder why the P can't make simple decisions. (And the J knows exactly which way the TP and paper towels should come over the roll.) All in all, the J can lend structure and stability to just about any situation, and this is a wonderful trait, as long as they remain open to allowing for inevitable change.

ISFJ, CHAKRAS & BALANCE

I will now acquaint you with suggested toolkits for the **ISFJ** that will include specific yoga postures, breathing practices (Pranayama) meditations, affirmations, and mudras (seals or 'hand yoga').

After an explanation of the 'toolkits' I have chosen to help enhance and maintain your natural strength as well as regain balance when necessary, there will be a short series of questions you can ask yourself to clarify just which energy field is most in need of attention.

Suggested Toolkits to Celebrate,
Nurture & Restore Balance:
Root Chakra, Sacral Chakra,
Solar Plexus Chakra

*(Depending on your particular life situation, ANY of the chakras may 'deserve' attention.
You can determine this by reviewing the questions found in each toolkit.)*

The combination of being a dominant Sensor ("team captain" of your type) along with a J lifestyle, (S-J) results in a structured, organized personality type. You are at your best when life is running in a predictable, systematic manner. You shine when your dependable nature is allowed to express itself and is appreciated by those in this realm of caring. Maintaining a balanced **ROOT CHAKRA** will enable you to share these gifts of orchestration in a healthy manner. This is also the flow you may choose to practice if you are perhaps going through a period of transition or much unexpected change.

On the other hand if you feel that you are being 'weighed down' and having a difficult time getting motivated, it's time to turn to the **SACRAL CHAKRA TOOLKIT**. The sacral chakra is all about flow, movement and the water element. It takes the solid foundation of the root chakra (earth element) and prepares the ground for the planting: seeds of creativity, newness and desire. We achieve these goals through motion, even if it's just a step at a time, opening our channels to the gifts of inspiration.

As a Feeler (your team 'co-captain'), if you are experiencing a sense depletion due to an enabling situation, you may find feelings of resentment rising up inside you. The combination of Feeling and Judging (F-J) can many times result in a sense of emotional obligation. (If THEY aren't going to be responsible enough to take care of themselves, I guess I need to step in...)

The **SOLAR PLEXUS CHAKRA TOOLKIT** can come to the rescue. When the heart energy field is weakened or drained, the need arises for building up feelings of confidence and self-esteem so that the playing field is again leveled. (Practicing flows to expand the Heart Chakra as this courage develops would be beneficial as well.)

All types need to be cognizant of the role that the throat chakra plays in our ability to communicate. The I-F will need to be wary of suppressing truth in the interest of not hurting anyone's feelings at the expense of their own health and personal truth.

Questions for the ISFJ to ask themselves to determine which Chakra to nurture:

1) "Do I feel connected and affirmed in my own right to have and to be?"

If YES, practice ROOT CHAKRA flows and meditations with the intention of not only enjoying your own sense of stability, but radiating this groundedness as a gift to others in your field of energy. If NO, practice ROOT CHAKRA toolkit offerings to help bring you back into a connection with the earth and a sense of grounding.

2) "Am I feeling stuck in a situation that is weighing me down and find myself taking on too much responsibility?"

If YES, practice SACRAL CHAKRA flows and meditations to bring motion and energy into your being. Keep your own desires and dreams in mind as you allow the motion to set you free.

3) *"Have I reached a point where I am sponge for other people's pain and feel unable to voice my frustration?"*

If YES, practice SOLAR PLEXUS CHAKRA flows and meditations to increase the confidence and vigor within yourself. This 'fire' will reignite feelings of personal power that are necessary not only to enable you to practice self-care (essential), but to continue to share love with others in your life from a healthy, balanced place.

As always, no matter which energy field we are currently engaging, it is important to hold your intention in both mind and heart and then be open to the inspiration that follows.

ENERGY TYPES

INFJ (Introverted-Intuitive-Feeling-Judger) - Robin Hood

$\mathcal{O}$kay, not that the INFJ will steal from the rich to give to the poor, but they WILL have a myriad of ideas about saving humanity that will be processed in a somewhat discreet and similar fashion. When an injustice is recognized, they will first look to the alternatives as far as what action needs to be initiated and then the actual process gets started. Maybe. It is imperative that the INFJ emerge from their possibility-abundant thought processes and put their Judger preference (closure) to work for them.

Being a Feeler as well as a Judger, tying up loose ends is indeed important to them, and as with most F-Js, they may have a tendency to tie them up just to avoid conflict or hurting someone. "Okay, all done. Let's move on." (But not really.) If they happen to be the one experiencing the bruised feelings, their dominant iNtuitive mode will quickly scan the many reasons for this rebuff. In the process, the level of pain could well escalate as their J bangs down the gavel on how wronged they have been. This whole scenario, by the way, could play out in total silence. You may only witness the fine streams of steam emerging from their ears as the 'injustice' gets tucked down within the heart. This is an area where most of us,

61

indeed Introverted-Feelers, should truly take heed. Pretending that an incident has not occurred or ignoring it will only lead to built-up frustration that will terminate in an eruption of emotion at some later point.

The INFJ can prove to be one of the best listeners you will ever encounter and will sincerely absorb what you are sharing with them. Because of this talent for being attentive to the outpourings and needs of others, they make excellent counselors, therapists and teachers, best in the realm of higher education. This, though, also escalates the necessity for them to vent their own feelings from time to time in a healthy, loving atmosphere, even if that be journaling. Otherwise they could end up on system overload attempting to administer 'healing waters to the thirsty' - from an empty well.

INFJs are probably some of the most 'generous contributors' to the world of self-help seminars and books sales on self- awareness. The typical NF penchant for figuring out "Who am I and why am I here?" will keep this genre of education well supported.

In intimate relationships, the INFJ will first circle the situation a bit like a lion taking stock of its prey, scrutinizing the whole scenario. As they become more trusting, the circle will diminish in size and they will move closer to the core. When they are finally convinced it's 'safe,' they will then be ready to invest heart and soul into the relationship. Being NFs (iNtuitive-Feelers) they will expect (if not demand) reciprocity of feelings, not necessarily through the spoken word, but actively shared nonetheless.

On the home front, things will normally appear quite orderly, that is until you open the closets and look under the beds. The J will want at least the appearance of a well organized house and yard, but there are far too many more globally important matters to attend to than dusting.

Compassionate, driven and on purpose... In the INFJ world, still waters run deep.

HIERARCHY OF FUNCTION ("Who's On First?")

The middle two letters of a person's type - our 'functions' - will equate to how we experience (perceive) reality and how we make our decisions. The 'authority' as to which of these processes occurs first will vary by type. There is an order we go through when accessing them and this is pretty much determined by the 'comfort zones' within our individual type.

We each have...
a DOMINANT FUNCTION (Team Captain)
an AUXILIARY FUNCTION (Co-captain)
a TERTIARY FUNCTION (Third at bat)
and an INFERIOR FUNCTION (Benchwarmer)

Of note, the Extravert (E) will 'share' their dominant process with the world and internalize their auxiliary. The Introvert (I) will do the opposite, keeping their most pre-ferred function internal and showing the world the 'next in command.'

This is the breakdown fo the INFJ:
DOMINANT (introverted) N
AUXILIARY (extraverted) F
TERTIARY (introverted) T
INFERIOR (extraverted) S

Type Preference by Letter for the INFJ:

E/I (Extraversion /Introversion): *How we are energized...* If you choose **Introversion** over Extraversion, you are usually most energized when spending quiet time alone or in the company of one or two close friends. You process things internally which Extraverts often find frustrating as they are not being kept up to date with minute by minute proceedings. If you want the most truthful, complete answer from an I, give them time to withdraw from the ruckus of the outer world and go within. Introverts also do not have the need to share their entire life story with people in line at the bank or sitting next to them on a plane. They are usually quite content to exist in their own universe until a need is felt to 'come out and play.' Now Introverts also need people, but being around too many people for too long a time can physically make them wither. As with any of the preferences, preservation of health means maintaining balance.

S/N (Sensing/iNtuition): *How we gather information...* This preference boils down to how we perceive reality, which is indeed a vital component in communication. If we are experiencing *different* realities, learning to see things through the eyes of the receiving party will enable us to share in a way that will be understood. Choosing **iNtuition** over Sensing indicates being engaged in the world of possibilities, trusting gut feelings over past experience, looking to the future vs. what is currently 'on the table,' and therefore not always being totally cognizant of what is going on right in front of one's nose. (e.g. walking right by something without seeing it if they aren't looking for it. And actually, sometimes even then). This is in contrast to the Sensor's comfort zone in the 'here and now' and trusting of five senses over conjecture.

T/F (Thinking/Feeling): *How we make our decisions...* If you choose **Feeling** over Thinking as your method of decision making, you tend to become embedded in the situation you are currently encountering. While we all practice both modes of determination, this arena will most often be a more comfortable fit for you. And though one will feel more natural, it is highly beneficial to learn to look at both sides of an issue, subjectively as well as objectively. In the world of the Feeler, this is where things like "constructive criticism" become an oxymoron. If you are critical of an F from any standpoint, you can almost be certain they will be hurt. One of the biggest gifts the MBTI® offers, is the understanding of *why* we process certain things the way we do. For example, in this situation, the Feeler could learn that yes, it is okay to decide with your heart, but don't forget to balance it out by taking a step back, removing yourself as if a bystander. Then take another look at the situation from this perspective. This is also helpful when dealing with Thinkers who may appear harsh or overly critical. Once it's understood that this is a decision making PROCESS, and not meant to be accusatory, these two preference types can come to much better understanding. (The same being true for the Thinker dealing with the Feeler: "Why do you take everything to heart?") In truth, as in all preference pairings, we can learn so much from one another.

J/P (Judging/Perceiving): *Our lifestyle...* Choosing **Judging** over Perceiving usually indicates a preference for closure, structure and lists. "Let's wrap it up" could be the motto of most Js. Open ends tend to make them uncomfortable. Now many times, especially for the Feeling-Judger, this could mean coming to closure just to avoid hurt feelings or any kind of conflict. (Which, depending on the situation, means you may end up having to deal with the scenario all over again.) This is in contrast to the P who prefers flexibility and leaving the door open until all options have been studied (or playing what I refer to as "ostrich." This entails putting your head in the ground and avoiding the fact that a decision even needs to be made.) Judgers like to live by a list and get a sense of achievement with crossing something off of that list. When living with a P, they may become critical if things aren't returned to their original place and also wonder why the P can't make simple decisions. (And the J knows exactly which way the TP and paper towels should come over the roll.) All in all, the J can lend structure and stability to just about any situation, and this is a wonderful trait, as long as they remain open to allowing for inevitable change

INFJ, CHAKRAS & BALANCE

I will now acquaint you with suggested toolkits for the **INFJ** that will include specific yoga postures, breathing practices (Pranayama) meditations, affirmations, and mudras (seals or 'hand yoga).

After an explanation of the 'toolkits' I have chosen to help enhance and maintain your natural strength as well as regain balance when necessary, there will be a short series of questions you can ask yourself to clarify just which energy field is most in need of attention.

Suggested Toolkits to Celebrate, Nurture & Restore Balance:
Third Eye Chakra, Root Chakra, Heart Chakra
(Depending on your particular life situation, ANY of the chakras may 'deserve' attention. You can determine this by reviewing the questions found in each toolkit.)

The 'team captain' for the INFJ, the iNtuitive perceiving function will be a realm of natural strength. In order to celebrate this process, I would recommend practicing the flow and meditation found in the **THIRD EYE CHAKRA** toolkit. Especially if you find yourself at a time in your life where dreams and 'gut feelings' are particularly strong and accurate, this flow will bring even further clarity to your path.

Now, it is important to recognize the tendency for a dominant N to also spend an inordinate amount of time in that 'interior castle of options,' especially considering that you tend to be energized through Introversion. In order to allow these ideas to blossom into more than just passing fancies, combining Third Eye Chakra flow with the tools found within the **ROOT CHAKRA** toolkit would give foundation to these dreams through the incorporation of stability and grounding.

The **THIRD EYE CHAKRA** toolkit will also be of benefit should you feel yourself UNABLE to access that normal myriad of ideas. You can 'rev it up' through a similar process, just focusing on a different intention. (For example, "I now open myself to new and beautiful inspirational ideas.")

Your 'co-captain,' the Feeling function, will also prove key in supporting these visions by bringing you into a decision-making mode.

As an iNtuitive Feeler (NF) there may be the propensity for over-extending yourself in the realm of rescuing. Narrowing the plethora of possibilities down to a manageable, concrete plan will streamline your intent. Practicing the flow and meditation found within the **HEART CHAKRA** toolkit should assist you in bringing clarity to what is truly most important.

All types need to be cognizant of the role that the throat chakra plays in our ability to communicate. The I-F will need to be wary of suppressing truth in the interest of not hurting anyone's feelings at the expense of their own health and personal truth.

Questions for the INFJ to ask themselves to determine which Chakra to nurture:

1) "Am I feeling energized and productive in relation to the beautiful possibilities in my life?"

If YES, practice THIRD EYE CHAKRA flows and meditations with the intention of honoring your innate gift of 'seeing' the vast playing field of options and alternatives. If NO, then turn also to this toolkit to reinspire those strengths.

2) "Am I feeling slightly overwhelmed (or even completely untethered) as to how to harness the many ideas and desires swirling within my mind?"

If YES, practice ROOT CHAKRA flows and meditations to bring those inspirations and intentions back down to earth. (As mentioned above, the combo of Third Eye and Root Chakra is pretty much always recommended, to capitalize on the idea process.)

3) *"Am I longing to put my project into action but experiencing a sense of confusion concerning who I can assist and how?"* And/or, *"Do I feel comfort in giving but have a difficult time receiving the same offers of generosity?"*

If YES, practice HEART CHAKRA flows and meditations to bring yourself into an authentic place within your own heart where a knowing will unfold and establish a framework for manifestation. (Affirm that you are centered and focused in targeting your vision.)

As always, no matter which energy field we are currently engaging, it is important to hold your intention in both mind and heart and then be open to the inspiration that follows.

ENERGY TYPES

INTJ (Introverted-iNtuitive-Thinking-Judger) - The Intellectual

*T*he INTJ makes wonderful use of the internal world of possibilities as they logically calculate how to implement these ideas, bring them to closure, and share their discovery with the world (perhaps). Many of the remarkable concepts being born of these intellectuals may seem to come about spontaneously when in actuality, they have been a work in progress that would not be shared until honed to their own perfectionist ideals.

The combination of iNtuition and Thinking (NT) can sometimes come across as cold or uncaring to the people in their lives. Combine this with introversion and the danger exists that fully inaccurate messages are being relayed. Still waters run deep and an understanding of Type can help to alleviate many falsely interpreted signals.

But once one gets beyond the aloof exterior of the INTJ, you will actually find someone who can not only be genuinely empathetic, but who will stand by you in your darkest hour. And it' s noteworthy to remember as in dealing with ALL Thinkers, this is just the label that represents a preference for objective decision-making and that they do indeed have feelings, too.

Curious and competitive, this type will dig deep to find answers and keep on digging until they do find them. If these 'answers' don't quite live up to their own expectations, they could be known to invent their own. Skepticism is an innate part of their make-up, so if you are presenting a project or an idea to an INTJ, be prepared for scrutiny.

Due to their perfectionist tendencies, (found in most NTs), they will attempt to achieve a degree of excellence in just about any endeavor they undertake, no matter the level of inherent life importance. And if the results don't live up to what they consider to be adequate, they can be quite tough on themselves. (That being said, those living and working with the INTJ may also feel a sense of responsibility for achieving levels of greatness due to expectations being met.)

When the INTJ encounters a reasonable amount of stress, their strengths are typically magnified in the quest for realizing a goal. This, by the way, is quite natural for all types. But equally true of all types, when the stress levels become unhealthy, the more underdeveloped preferences may appear on the horizon and not always in the most attractive manner. For the INTJ, this could appear as overly-detailed conduct (i.e. picky) and possible martyr-like behavior, as the Sensing and Feeling sides of their persona are being tweaked.

The INTJ may not always have patience for those wearing their heart on their sleeve and therefore, when dealing with a situation where much emotion is involved, may have the tendency to sweep the sentiments under the rug to attend to 'more logical' issues.

In the realm of romance, their introverted, independent nature will most likely appear as a laid-back stance, as they allow themselves to digest the potential repercussions involved in a possible partnership. Most likely turned-off by flightiness, the INTJ will find harmony when paired with an intellectual equal, where the conversations are as meaningful as the love life and a penchant for adventure is part of the package.

From a vocational standpoint, the NT can almost always be found in an arena that not only offers a challenge but one that includes futuristic, cutting-edge philosophies. If 'stuck' in a job that is too predictable, it will be endured under great duress or left all together. You will find INTJs in professions such as consulting, teaching (university level), writing and any area where they can use their minds to contribute to the world in an innovative fashion.

Independent, philosophical, and forward-thinking, the INTJ forges many a path that brings wide-spread benefit to all.

Type Preference by Letter for the INTJ:

E/I (Extraversion /Introversion): *How we are energized...* If you choose **Introversion** over Extraversion, you are usually most energized when spending quiet time alone or in the company of one or two close friends. You process things internally which Extraverts often find frustrating as they are not being kept up to date with minute by minute proceedings. If you want the most truthful, complete answer from an I, give them time to withdraw from the ruckus of the outer world and go within. Introverts also do not have the need to share their entire life story with people in line at the bank or sitting next to them on a plane. They are usually quite content to exist in their own universe until a need is felt to 'come out and play.'

HIERARCHY OF FUNCTION ("Who's On First?")

The middle two letters of a person's type - our 'functions' - will equate to how we experience (perceive) reality and how we make our decisions. The 'authority' as to which of these processes occurs first will vary by type. There is an order we go through when accessing them and this is pretty much determined by the 'comfort zones' of our individual type.

We each have...
a DOMINANT FUNCTION (Team Captain)
an AUXILIARY FUNCTION (Co-captain)
a TERTIARY FUNCTION (Third at bat)
and an INFERIOR FUNCTION (Benchwarmer)

Of note, the Extravert (E) will 'share' their dominant process with the world and internalize their auxiliary. The Introvert (I) will do the opposite, keeping their most preferred function internal and showing the world the 'next in command.'

This is the breakdown fo the INTJ:
DOMINANT (introverted) N
AUXILIARY (extraverted) T
TERTIARY (introverted) F
INFERIOR (extraverted) S

E/I continued...

Now Introverts also need people, but being around too many people for too long a time can physically make them wither. As with all preferences, preservation of health means maintaining balance.

S/N (Sensing/iNtuition): *How we gather information...* This preference boils down to how we take in information, a vital component in communication. If we are experiencing *different* realities, learning to see things through the eyes of the receiving party will enable us to share in a way that will be understood. Choosing **iNtuition** over Sensing indicates being engaged in the world of possibilities, trusting gut feelings over past experience, looking to the future vs. what is currently 'on the table,' and therefore not always being totally cognizant of what is going on right in front of one's nose. (e.g. walking right by something without seeing it if they aren't looking for it. And actually, sometimes even then). This is in contrast to the Sensor's comfort zone in the 'here and now' and trusting of five senses over conjecture.

T/F (Thinking/Feeling): *How we make our decisions...* These are both rational means of decision-making but one will almost always offer a much more natural approach. When **Thinking** is preferred over Feeling (again please recall that these are Jungian terms and don't indicate that we don't all do both) the decisions will be more from the head than the heart i.e. the T tends to take an objective stance apart from the situation vs becoming embedded in the process. While we all practice both modes of determination and one will be more natural, it is highly beneficial to learn to look at both sides of an issue, subjectively as well as objectively. In the world of the Feeler, this is where things like "constructive criticism" become an oxymoron. If you are critical of an F from any standpoint, you can almost be certain they will be hurt. One of the biggest gifts the MBTI® offers, is the understanding of *why* we process certain things the way we do. For example, in this situation, the Feeler could learn that yes, it is okay to decide with your heart, but don't forget to balance it out by taking a step back and viewing the situation from the perspective of an observer. This is also helpful when dealing with Thinkers who may appear harsh or overly critical. Once it's understood that this is a decision making

PROCESS, and not meant to be accusatory, these two preference types can come to much better understanding. (The same being true for the Thinker dealing with the Feeler: "Why do you take everything to heart?") In truth, as in all preference pairings, we can learn so much from one another.

J/P (Judging/Perceiving): *Our lifestyle...* Choosing **Judging** over Perceiving usually indicates a preference for closure, structure and lists. "Let's wrap it up" could be the motto of most Js. Open ends tend to make them uncomfortable. Now many times, especially for the Feeling-Judger, this could mean coming to closure just to avoid hurt feelings or any kind of conflict. (Which, depending on the situation, means you may end up having to deal with the scenario all over again.) This is in contrast to the P who prefers flexibility and leaving the door open until all options have been studied (or playing what I refer to as "ostrich." This entails putting your head in the ground and avoiding the fact that a decision even needs to be made.) Judgers like to live by a list and get a sense of achievement with crossing something off of that list. When living with a P, they may become critical if things aren't returned to their original place and also wonder why the P can't make simple decisions. (And the J knows exactly which way the TP and paper towels should come over the roll.) All in all, the J can lend structure and stability to just about any situation, and this is a wonderful trait, as long as they remain open to allowing for inevitable change.

INTJ, CHAKRAS & BALANCE

I will now acquaint you with suggested toolkits for the **INTJ** that will include specific yoga postures, breathing practices (Pranayama) meditations, affirmations, and mudras (seals or 'hand yoga).

After an explanation of the 'toolkits' I have chosen to help enhance and maintain your natural strength as well as regain balance when necessary, there will be a short series of questions you can ask yourself to clarify just which energy field is most in need of attention.

Suggested Toolkits to Celebrate, Nurture & Restore Balance:
Third Eye Chakra, Root Chakra, Heart Chakra

(Depending on your particular life situation, ANY of the chakras may 'deserve' attention. You can determine this by reviewing the questions found in each toolkit.)

The 'team captain' for the INTJ, the iNtuitive perceiving function will be a realm of natural strength. In order to celebrate this process, I would recommend practicing the flow and meditation found in the **THIRD EYE CHAKRA** toolkit. Especially if you find yourself at a time in your life where dreams and 'gut feelings' are particulary strong and accurate, this will help bring even further clarity to your path.

Now, it is important to recognize the tendency for a dominant N to also spend an inordinate amount of time in that 'interior castle of options,' especially considering that you tend to be energized through Introversion. In order to allow these ideas to blossom into more than just passing fancies, combining Third Eye Chakra flow with the tools found within the **ROOT CHAKRA** toolkit would give foundation to these dreams through the accessing of stablity and grounding.

The **THIRD EYE CHAKRA** toolkit will also be of benefit should you feel yourself UNABLE to acces that normal myriad of ideas.

You can 'rev it up' through a similar process, just focusing on a different intention. (For example, "I now open myself to new and beautiful inspirational ideas.")

Your 'co-captain,' the Thinking function, will also prove key in supporting these visions by bringing you into a decision-making mode. As an iNtuitive Thinker (NT), though, you may need to spend some time getting in tune with the essence of what you are creating vs the perfection of the final outcome. Practicing the flow and meditation found within the **HEART CHAKRA** toolkit should assist you in bringing clarity to what is truly most important.

All types need to be cognizant of the role that the throat chakra plays in our ability to communicate. The I-T will need to be wary of avoiding issues because they feel 'uncomfortable' or 'none of my business.' But if areas of discomfort become suppressed rather than expressed, you may find that your health and emotional stability suffer as a result of not speaking your truth.

Questions for the INTJ to ask themselves to determine which Chakra to nurture:

1) "Am I feeling energized and productive in relation to the beautiful possibilities in my life?"

If YES, practice THIRD EYE CHAKRA flows and meditations with the intention of honoring your innate gifts of 'seeing' the vast playing field of options and alternatives. If NO, then turn also to this toolkit to reinspire those strengths.

2) *"Am I feeling slightly overwhelmed (or even completely untethered) as to how to harness the many ideas and desires swirling within my mind?"*

If YES, practice ROOT CHAKRA flows and meditations to bring bring those inspirations and intentions back down to earth. (As mentioned above, the combo of Third Eye and Root Chakra is pretty much always recommended to capitalize on the idea process.)

3) *"Am I finding myself spending too much time in arenas that are not fully encompassing the passion behind my vision?"*

If YES, practice HEART CHAKRA flows and meditations to bring yourself into an authentic place within your own heart where a knowing will unfold and establish a framework for manifestation. (Affirm that you are centered and focused in targeting your vision.)

As always, no matter which energy field we are currently engaging, it is important to hold your intention in both mind and heart and then be open to the inspiration that follows.

ENERGY TYPES

ISTP (Introverted-Sensing-Thinking-Perceiver)
- It Is What It Is

$\mathcal{H}$ave you ever known anyone who is drawn to take something apart just to see how it works? And then after satisfying their curiousity, it is reconstructed to work even more smoothly than originally designed (even minus the two parts that didn't get reassembled)? You could very well be watching an ISTP in action. Dominant (introverted) Thinkers (Ts), the logic of why something functions the way it does can be quite provocative. Add the Sensing-Perceiving nature to the mix and the process becomes an ongoing way of life. They are processing the events, circumstances and details evolving around them in real time. Picture a batter in a batting cage awaiting the next ball. Bring it on, I'm ready for you!

As with most Sensing-Perceivers, the ISTP is quite adept at handling crisis situations. Their innate comfort in tackling moment-to-moment developments proves itself as well in emergencies.

This knack for rolling with the punches equips the ISTP with a versatile outlook on life in both its joy as well as its challenges. The Thinking team captain keeps them in an objective frame of mind, thus endowing this type with a penchant for realism. If things get too theoretical or mushy, it's time to move on. Just the facts, please. Not that they don't have feelings, it's just not a realm that they feel drawn to explore and therefore are not especially comfortable with, either.

Those around them may, though, be perplexed at times when trying to pinpoint just what is going on inside the ISTP. Their Introversion takes this reality-based outlook to a place that is private and not often presented to the world at large. Because of this, they could be misread in their intentions, as needs and wants may go unexpressed.

The ISTP can become bored if they experience a lack of stimulation and will hastily move on to a new project if this ennui sets in. The caveat here is that the current enterprise being worked on may never come to completion. They, on the other hand, may feel that they are making great strides in accomplishing a number of things, as they have twelve ventures going simultaneously. Again, key here is the matter of fulfillment. The ISTP could take some pointers from Judging (J) comrades in realizing the importance of follow through. Try to share this, though, as if it was their own idea and you will make more progress.

The ISTP under stress may initially appear even more introverted and focused on matters at hand. But should the stress escalate, as with most types, you could witness a flip-flop in what would be considered 'normal' behavior for their type. In this case, issues that may have initially appeared just annoying could take on importance of global implication and need to be rectified NOW. This should be a red flag in any case.

Intimate relationships may not be high on the agenda of this type, as commitment could carry rather 'long-term' implications and that is not the most ideal playing field for the ISTP. When they do decide to get involved, it will be a seriously regarded undertaking. However, it would be wise to take into account that if greener pastures avail themselves, it would not be acharacteristic for them to wish you well and move on.

Careerwise, the ISTP will likely find the highest degree of satisfaction in areas that speak to their love of action, flexibility and tangible results. Construction, extreme sports, mechanical arenas, firefighting, police or military arenas are areas that come to mind.

Spontaneous, technical and risk-taking, the ISTP adds adventure and objectivity to our world.

Type Preference by Letter for the ISTP:

E/I (Extraversion /Introversion): *How we are energized...* If you choose **Introversion** over Extraversion, you are usually most energized when spending quiet time alone or in the company of one or two close friends. You process things internally which Extraverts often find frustrating as they are not being kept up to date with minute by minute proceedings. If you want the most truthful, complete answer from an I, give them time to withdraw from the ruckus of the outer world and go within. Introverts also do not have the need to share their entire life story with people in line at the bank or sitting next to them on a plane. They are usually quite content to exist in their own universe until a need is felt to 'come out and play.' Now Introverts also need people, but being around too many people for too long a time can physically make them wither. As with all preferences, preservation of health means maintaining balance.

HIERARCHY OF FUNCTION ("Who's On First?")

The middle two letters of a person's type - our 'functions' - will equate to how we experience (perceive) reality and how we make our decisions. The 'authority' as to which of these processes occurs first will vary by type. There is an order we go through when accessing them and this is pretty much determined by the 'comfort zones' of our individual type.

We each have...
a DOMINANT FUNCTION (Team Captain)
an AUXILIARY FUNCTION (Co-captain)
a TERTIARY FUNCTION (Third at bat)
and an INFERIOR FUNCTION (Benchwarmer)

Of note, the Extravert (E) will 'share' their dominant process with the world and internalize their auxiliary. The Introvert (I) will do the opposite, keeping their most preferred function internal and showing the world the 'next in command.'

This is the breakdown fo the ISTP:
DOMINANT (introverted) T
AUXILIARY (extraverted) S
TERTIARY (introverted) N
INFERIOR (introverted) F

Type Preference by Letter continued...

S/N (Sensing/iNtuition): *How we perceive reality...* This preference boils down to how take in information, a vital component in communication. If we are experiencing *different* realities, learning to see things through the eyes of the receiving party will enable us to share in a way that will be understood. If you choose **Sensing** over iNtuition, you are probably very engaged in the world of detail, the past and day-to-day experience. Living in the present and in the tactile world of the five senses - i.e. what you see, hear, taste, smell and touch - is your reality and you are quite attuned to your environment. (This in comparison to the iNtuitive who resides in the realm of possibilities, trusts 'gut feelings' over past experience, is future-oriented and not always cognizant of what is going on in the physical world. They tend to live beyond the 5 senses.) Being practical and dealing with 'what is' as opposed to 'what could be' are key attributes of the Sensing Type. The S may also take things quite literally which the N should keep in mind when sharing information as miscommunication *could* run rampant. ("You SAID be here on the hour... but you DIDN'T say which one!") All in all, they can make great partners, but understanding the different modes of perception is essential.

T/F (Thinking/Feeling): *How we make our decisions...* These are both rational means of decision-making but one will almost always offer a much more natural approach. When **Thinking** is preferred over Feeling (again please recall that these are Jungian terms and don't indicate that we don't all do both) the decisions will be more from the head than the heart i.e. the T tends to take an objective stance apart from the situation vs becoming embedded in the process. While we all practice both modes of determination and one will be more natural, it is highly beneficial to learn to look at both sides of an issue, subjectively as well as objectively. In the world of the Feeler, this is where things like "constructive criticism" become an oxymoron. If you are critical of an F from any standpoint, you can almost be certain they will be hurt. One of the biggest gifts the MBTI® offers, is the understanding of *why* we process certain things the way we do. For example, in this situation, the Feeler could learn that yes, it is okay to decide with your heart, but don't forget to balance it out by taking a step back and viewing the situation from the perspective of an observer. This is also helpful when dealing with

Thinkers who may appear harsh or overly critical. Once it's understood that this is a decision making PROCESS, and not meant to be accusatory, these two preference types can come to much better understanding. (The same being true for the Thinker dealing with the Feeler: "Why do you take everything to heart?") In truth, as in all preference pairings, we can learn so much from one another.

J/P (Judging/Perceiving): *Our lifestyle...* Choosing **Perceiving** over Judging will usually result in being into open ends, spontaneity, and flexibility. (vs J closure, list making and structure). This could lead to a lot of unfinished projects as something gets started and the P is sidetracked by something 'more important.' The P probably doesn't get too ruffled when plans change and could even be known to change them, just to shake things up a little. The natural leanings of the P could lead to viewing endless 'what ifs' when trying to come to closure, resulting in procrastination and not surprisingly, tardiness. Incorporating a little of the the J's love of schedules could assist in being more organized. Once again the AWARENESS is invaluable. Many times we can be totally oblivious to certain personality characteristics until they are pointed out in tangible form. But remember, Type should never used as an excuse; for example, "It's okay for me to be involved in 12 different projects (and so who cares about completion), I'm a P." That's a no-go 'cause if you are aware of being a P, then you need to take the responsibility and work on the potential stumbling blocks associated with that preference. So there.

ISTP, CHAKRAS & BALANCE

I will now acquaint you with suggested toolkits for the **ISTP** that will include specific yoga postures, breathing practices (Pranayama) meditations, affirmations, and mudras (seals or 'hand yoga).

After an explanation of the 'toolkits' I have chosen to help enhance and maintain your natural strength as well as regain balance when necessary, there will be a short series of questions you can ask yourself to clarify just which energy field is most in need of attention.

Suggested Toolkits to Celebrate, Nurture & Restore Balance:
Solar Plexus Chakra, Root Chakra, Heart Chakra

(Depending on your particular life situation, ANY of the chakras may 'deserve' attention. You can determine this by reviewing the questions found in each toolkit.)

The dominant Thinking function of the ISTP will serve you well when looking to your 'inner power' to achieve a goal or complete a mission, whether that be running the mile under 5 minutes or leading troops into battle. To celebrate this innate preference, spending time in the **SOLAR PLEXUS TOOLKIT** will focus that energy on the 'sun within' and feelings of courage. Should you feel depleted regarding the confidence necessary to move forward towards a goal, this is also a good place to start to rekindle the fire.

Maintaining a balanced **ROOT CHAKRA** is also important, because your love of change and action can sometimes play havoc with your ability to commit or come to closure. This toolkit will enable you to incorporate the structure you may need to stay grounded and stable.

As you typically experience your comfort zone when introspectively living in the logic of the moment, you could find that your heart chakra is not getting the attention it needs. This could occur from two different perspectives: Allowing yourself to accept and appreci-

87

ate the love and attention being offered you or in your ability to share love, compassion and appreciation with the others in your life. Spending time in the **HEART CHAKRA TOOLKIT** can offer you the balance that will keep the relationship with yourself as well others in a healthy state.

All types need to be cognizant of the role that the throat chakra plays in our ability to communicate. The I-T will need to be wary of avoiding issues because they feel 'uncomfortable' or 'none of my business.' But if areas of discomfort become suppressed rather than expressed, you may find that your health and emotional stability suffer as a result of not speaking your truth.

Questions for the ISTP to ask themselves to determine which Chakra to nurture:

1) "Am I feeling motivated and inspired to tackle projects that are coming my way?"

If YES, practice SOLAR PLEXUS CHAKRA flows and meditations with the intention of marching forward with confidence. If NO, practice SOLAR PLEXUS CHAKRA toolkit offerings to help bring you back into your natural love of adventure.

2) "Am I feeling unable to make commitments or bring about necessary closure that will bring structure to my life plans?"

If YES, practice ROOT CHAKRA flows and meditations to connect you to the earth element of rootedness and stability. Allow that fertile ground to be a foundation for the seeds of your creativity.

3) "Do I feel blocked when it comes to giving and receiving love and affection in my life?"

If YES, practice HEART CHAKRA flows and meditations to increase your ability to be open to self-love and care as well as the warmth that others in your life desire to share with you.

As always, no matter which energy field we are currently engaging, it is important to hold your intention in both mind and heart and then be open to the inspiration that follows.

ENERGY TYPES

ISFP (Introverted-Sensing-Feeling-Perceiver) - There's No Time Like the Present

$\mathcal{P}$rivate, caring and 'in-the-moment.' the ISFP has a certain sensitivity that may not always be readily apparent, though Feeling is the 'captain of their team.' It also happens to be an introverted function, so the world is more aware of the realistic bent represented by their extraverted Sensing co-captain. Combine this with the Perceiving preference, and a sometimes 'fly by the seat of your pants' inclination is the result. Taking things too seriously should be reserved for death and taxes.

This type finds a distinct solace in nature and though the activity may vary, being outside doing SOMETHING will bring a sense of peace. (And leave the watch at home.)

As with many types who share the letters S and P, they will be quick to react and quite capable in an emergency situation. Their proclivity for being in the present moment will aid them in taking care of what needs to be done RIGHT NOW (though after the fact, their Feeling preference may then take over and lead to some post-event anxiety). This being said, while many types can yield to an addictive nature for a myriad of reasons, the ISFP may have a more than average chance for developing substance dependencies. The I-F (Introverted-Feeling) aspect of the personality could have the tendency to promote the avoidance of painful life experiences. As they get tucked down deep inside, the antidote of choice for dealing with the pain may be to subdue it with some sort of numbing elixir.

If you wish to share something of real importance with an ISFP, my suggestion would be to put it in writing. If shared verbally, there is a chance it will enter one ear and exit the other without being totally assimilated. (This is actually a good thing to keep in mind when dealing with Introverts in general. By sharing written correspondence, they will have the time to digest the message without having to respond off the cuff. This translates into a much better chance of really communicating.)

In an intimate relationship, the ISFP will be cautious yet expectant. If it 'feels' right, they may just jump right in, but all the while holding their breath. If it pans out as expected, great! Exhale! If it takes a wrong turn, they may just hole up for a while and lick their wounds or find some tedious activity to take their mind off of the outcome. In the instance of success, however, they will prove to be caring, loving partners, though not always as expressive as might prove necessary for an open exchange of ideas. A reserved makeup could prevent them from sharing some of the more personal things about themselves either to prevent being hurt down the line or sometimes just in avoidance of deeper self-examination and its repercussions.

Under a heavy amount of stress you may witness the emergence of a completely altered persona, as the analytical nature of the "benchwarmer" Thinking function makes itself known, and probably not in an optimal manner. The laid back P will display some very atypically regimented behavior, most especially if they themselves or a loved one is being morally wronged. In cases of more minor daily stresses, you could also find them establishing a comfortable routine so that at least SOMETHING in their life is predictable e.g. "Monday is taco night."

In the workplace, the ISFP will usually be happiest when able to work at their own pace without being boxed in. In a restrictive environment, such as an office cubicle, their energy will have a tendency to take a distinct nosedive, particularly if they are subjected to the comings and goings of a variety of fellow office mates, phone calls, and... the dreaded meeting! Landscaping, athletics, oceanagraphy, ranch work, 'green' related business ventures - anything that allows them to take advantage of a natural setting in a less than structured setting would be balm to the heart of this type. If an outdoor environment is not a possibility, then a close follow up would be a small to medium-sized business where they can have a say regarding their schedule and work requirements and are not required to present to groups.

Discreet and a 'bit' noncommital, the ISFP offers the world a heart filled with compassion and a zest for the beauty found on this beautiful planet.

Type Preference by Letter for the ISFP:

E/I (Extraversion /Introversion): *How we are energized...* If you choose **Introversion** over Extraversion, you are usually most energized when spending quiet time alone or in the company of one or two close friends. You process things internally which Extraverts often find frustrating as they are not being kept up to date with

HIERARCHY OF FUNCTION ("Who's On First?")

The middle two letters of a person's type - our 'functions' - will equate to how we experience (perceive) reality and how we make our decisions. The 'authority' as to which of these processes occurs first will vary by type. There is an order we go through when accessing them and this is pretty much determined by the 'comfort zones' of our individual type.

We each have...
a DOMINANT FUNCTION (Team Captain)
an AUXILIARY FUNCTION (Co-captain)
a TERTIARY FUNCTION (Third at bat)
and an INFERIOR FUNCTION (Benchwarmer)

Of note, the Extravert (E) will 'share' their dominant process with the world and internalize their auxiliary. The Introvert (I) will do the opposite, keeping their most preferred function internal and showing the world the 'next in command.'

This is the breakdown fo the ISFP:
DOMINANT (introverted) F
AUXILIARY (extraverted) S
TERTIARY (introverted) N
INFERIOR (extraverted) T

E/I continued...

minute by minute proceedings. If you want the most truthful, complete answer from an I, give them time to withdraw from the ruckus of the outer world and go within. Introverts also do not have the need to share their entire life story with people in line at the bank or sitting next to them on a plane. They are usually quite content to exist in their own universe until a need is felt to 'come out and play.' Now Introverts also need people, but being around too many people for too long a time can physically make them wither. As with all preferences, preservation of health means maintaining balance.

S/N (Sensing/iNtuition): *How we perceive reality...* This preference boils down to how we take in information, a vital component in communication. If we are experiencing *different* realities, learning to see things through the eyes of the receiving party will enable us to share in a way that will be understood. If you choose **Sensing** over iNtuition, you are probably very engaged in the world of detail, the past and day-to-day experience. Living in the present and in the tactile world of the five senses - i.e. what you see, hear, taste, smell and touch - is your reality and you are quite attuned to your environment. (This in comparison to the iNtuitive who resides in the realm of possibilities, trusts 'gut feelings' over past experience, is future-oriented and not always cognizant of what is going on in the physical world. They tend to live beyond the 5 senses.) Being practical and dealing with 'what is' as opposed to 'what could be' are key attributes of the Sensing Type. The S may also take things quite literally which the N should keep in mind when sharing information as miscommunication *could* run rampant. ("You SAID be here on the hour... but you DIDN'T say which one!") All in all, they can make great partners, but understanding the different modes of perception is essential.

T/F (Thinking/Feeling): *How we make our decisions...* If you choose **Feeling** over Thinking as your method of decision making, you tend to become embedded in the situation you are currently encountering. While we all practice both modes of determination, this arena will most often be a more comfortable fit for you. And though one will feel more natural, it is highly beneficial to learn to look at both sides of an issue, subjectively as well as objectively. In the world of the Feeler, this is where things like "constructive criticism" become an oxymoron. If you are critical of an F from any standpoint, you can almost be certain they will be hurt. One of the biggest gifts the MBTI® offers, is the understanding of *why* we process certain things the way we do. For example, in this situation, the Feeler could learn that yes, it is okay to decide with your heart, but don't forget to balance it out by taking a step back and viewing the situation from the perspective of an observer. This is also helpful when dealing with Thinkers who may appear harsh or overly critical. Once it's understood that this is a decision making PROCESS, and not meant to be accusatory, these two preference types can come to much better understanding. (The same being true for the Thinker dealing with the Feeler: "Why do you take everything to heart?") In truth, as in all preference pairings, we can learn so much

J/P (Judging/Perceiving): *Our lifestyle...* Choosing **Perceiving** over Judging will usually result in being into open ends, spontaneity, and flexibility. (vs J closure, list making and structure). This could lead to a lot of unfinished project as something gets started and the P is sidetracked by something 'more important.' The P probably doesn't get too ruffled when plans change and could even be known to change them, just to shake things up a little. The natural leanings of the P could lead to viewing endless 'what ifs' when trying to come to closure, resulting in procrastination and not surprisingly, tardiness. Incorporating a little of the the J's love of schedules could assist in being more organized. Once again the AWARENESS is invaluable. Many times we can be totally oblivious to certain personality characteristics until they are pointed out in tangible form. But remember, Type should never be used as an excuse; for example, "It's okay for me to be involved in 12 different projects (and so who cares about completion), I'm a P." That's a no-go 'cause if you are aware of being a P, then you need to take the responsibility and work on the potential stumbling blocks associated with that preference. So there.

ISFP AND CHAKRA BALANCE

I will now acquaint you with suggested toolkits for the **ISFP** that will include specific yoga postures, breathing practices (Pranayama) meditations, affirmations, and mudras (seals or 'hand yoga).

After an explanation of the 'toolkits' I have chosen to help enhance and maintain your natural strength as well as regain balance when necessary, there will be a short series of questions you can ask yourself to clarify just which energy field is most in need of attention.

Suggested Toolkits to Celebrate, Nurture & Restore Balance: *Heart Chakra, Root Chakra, Solar Plexus Chakra*

(Depending on your particular life situation, ANY of the chakras may 'deserve' attention. You can determine this by reviewing the questions found in each toolkit.)

As a dominant Feeler ("team captain" of your type) the heart chakra will be your home playing field. When life is flowing along in a healthy state, the **HEART CHAKRA TOOLKIT** is where you can go to not only help maintain that balance, but to celebrate your gifts of empathy, compassion and heart-based leadership.

This is also the flow you may choose to practice if you ask yourself the question, "Am I feeling depleted?" and the answer is 'yes.' This could be in cases of going through a period of grief or having given so much of yourself due to life circumstances that you find yourself needing a dose of heart chakra nourishment. This will allow you to open up both sides of the heart - able to give, but also able to receive and keep the energy circulating.

97

Though the ISFP finds solace in nature, you can live so fully in the moment, flitting here and there, that your feet don't touch the ground anymore. In the interest of reeling you back into to the world of matter, spending time in the **ROOT CHAKRA TOOL-KIT** can bring you back to earth. This chakra is key in establishing the roots that provide stability and a right to be here, thereby removing the fear that can enter our being when we feel less than secure. Including a morning run or walk each day or just being out in nature and feeling your footfall on the earth also has a tremendously grounding influence.

If you are feeling depleted and in need of revving up your levels of confidence, turning to the **SOLAR PLEXUS TOOLKIT** is highly recommended. When we feel weakened or drained, we need to build up feelings of courage and self-esteem so that the playing field is leveled once again and decisions are made from a place of true inner power.

All types need to be cognizant of the role that the throat chakra plays in our ability to communicate. The I-F will need to be wary of suppressing truth in the interest of not hurting anyone's feelings - at the expense of their own health and personal truth.

Questions for the ISFP to ask themselves to determine which Chakra to nurture:

1) *"Am I in a position where my heart is leading the way and I feel strong and giving?"*

If YES, practice HEART CHAKRA TOOLKIT flows to maintain

this sense of heart-felt leadership. If NO, due to depletion through grief or inability to receive the love you deserve, turn to this toolkit as well.

2) *"Am I finding myself jumping haphazardly from one thing to another and therefore experiencing a loss of stability?*

If YES, turn to the ROOT CHAKRA TOOLKIT to reestabish your connection to the grounding of the earth element.

3) *"Are feelings of low self worth or loss of confidence keeping me from moving forward and achieving my goals?"*

If YES, practice SOLAR PLEXUS CHAKRA flows and meditations to increase the confidence and vigor within yourself. This 'fire' will reignite feelings of personal power that are necessary, not only to enable you to practice self-care, but to continue to share love with others in your life from a healthy, balanced place.

As always, no matter which energy field we are currently engaging, it is important to hold your intention in both mind and heart and then be open to the inspiration that follows.

ENERGY TYPES

INFP (Introverted Intuitive Feeling Perceiver) - Joan/John of Arc

As dominant Feelers, the INFP is quite in tune with the state of the world around them and where there might appear to be a need of any kind. This, though, is an internal process and what those around them will most likely first recognize will be the myriad of ideas that are being articulated, should they choose to share them. As Introverts, many of these intentions may remain in the realm of imagination. Then add the Perceiving function to boot and they may never actually see the light of day!

They are, in any case, driven by a strong set of inner values and strive to serve in idealistic ways. Outer appearances may suggest an easygoing nature, but if you step on the toes of one of these ideals, look out. There is power behind the nonchalant exterior. (Picture a mother lion protecting her cub.)

As a typical NF, they do have a need to please those with whom they are living or working, this for a two-fold reason. Not only do they enjoy giving of themselves, but they also abhor conflict, so better to keep everyone happy rather than cause waves. If there is a need to discuss a particular issue that is causing underlying friction, their Introversion could cause them to suppress what would often be better off shared. This is a due to the fact that those feelings will indeed rear their head at some point and when they finally do, it could result in a major (and what seems to appear as out-of-the-blue) outburst.

INFPs have quite high standards and while this might produce quality work, it can also lead to procrastination and self-criticism if the project isn't holding up to their escalated expectations. This is difficult enough when working on individual undertakings, but put them in a group venture and the dynamics could shift quite suddenly if everyone is not pulling their weight up to INFP standards.

As mentioned earlier, procrastination can be a hindrance in the forward motion of this type. As an Intuitive-Perceiver, the possibilities can seem endless when making a decision. Just a concrete knowledge that this could be the case will sometimes spur them on to try practicing more J behavior (i.e. lists, calendars, etc) but having a good J friend to keep them on their timely toes might be practical, too, as this tendency can lead to difficulty being punctual as well.

Under extreme stress, the INFP could be easily mistaken for a much more extraverted, detail-oriented type, sharing in a possibly not so demure manner just what they consider the facts of the situation. As with all types, taking a few deep breaths when under more than a healthy amount of stress is highly recommended.

In the romantic scheme of things, the INFP is quite discerning, allowing a situation to fully develop before throwing their heart over the fence. Especially if they have experienced a previous heartbreak or two, the footing will be very tentative until the partner in question has passed the litmus test. Once the exam is complete, however, the INFP will prove to be a dedicated 'significant other,' sometimes actually going overboard in their enthusiasm to please. One point of contention might be their reticence to talk about their innermost feelings, especially if it would convey a less than positive message. So if you are partnered with an INFP, most especially if you are another

Introvert, making the time to share what's going on internally could sometimes save a relationship.

In the work arena, the INFP will most likely find themselves in some type of service profession, perhaps in a counseling mode (one on one) or as a behind-the-scenes go-to person for fundraisers or non-profits. Writing is also heavily favored for this type as many do enjoy expressing themselves through the written word.

The INFP: idealistic, artistic and ready to make a difference in the world.

HIERARCHY OF FUNCTION ("Who's On First?")

The middle two letters of a person's type - our 'functions' - will equate to how we experience (perceive) reality and how we make our decisions. The 'authority' as to which of these processes occurs first will vary by type. There is an order we go through when accessing them and this is pretty much determined by the 'comfort zones' of our individual type.

We each have...
a DOMINANT FUNCTION (Team Captain)
an AUXILIARY FUNCTION (Co-captain)
a TERTIARY FUNCTION (Third at bat)
and an INFERIOR FUNCTION (Benchwarmer)

Of note, the Extravert (E) will 'share' their dominant process with the world and internalize their auxiliary. The Introvert (I) will do the opposite, keeping their most preferred function internal and showing the world the 'next in command.'

This is the breakdown fo the INFP:
DOMINANT (introverted) F
AUXILIARY (extraverted) N
TERTIARY (introverted) S
INFERIOR (extraverted) T

Type Preference by Letter for the INFP:

E/I (Extraversion /Introversion): *How we are energized...* If you choose **Introversion** over Extraversion, you are usually most energized when spending quiet time alone or in the company of one or two close friends. You process things internally which Extraverts often find frustrating as they are not being kept up to date with minute by minute proceedings. If you want the most truthful, complete answer from an I, give them time to withdraw from the ruckus of the outer world and go within. Introverts also do not have the need to share their entire life story with people in line at the bank or sitting next to them on a plane. They are usually quite content to exist in their own universe until a need is felt to 'come out and play.' Now Introverts also need people, but being around too many people for too long a time can physically make them wither. As with all preferences, preservation of health means maintaining balance.

S/N (Sensing/iNtuition): *How we gather information...* This preference boils down to how we take in information, a vital component in communication. If we are experiencing *different* realities, learning to see things through the eyes of the receiving party will enable us to share in a way that will be understood. Choosing **iNtuition** over Sensing indicates being engaged in the world of possibilities, trusting gut feelings over past experience, looking to the future vs. what is currently 'on the table,' and therefore not always being totally cognizant of what is going on right in front of one's nose. (e.g. walking right by something without seeing it if they aren't looking for it. And actually, sometimes even then). This is in contrast to the Sensor's comfort zone in the 'here and now' and trusting of five senses over conjecture.

T/F (Thinking/Feeling): *How we make our decisions...* If you choose

Feeling over Thinking as your method of decision making, you tend to become embedded in the situation you are currently encountering. While we all practice both modes of determination, this arena will most often be a more comfortable fit for you. And though one will feel more natural, it is highly beneficial to learn to look at both sides of an issue, subjectively as well as objectively. In the world of the Feeler, this is where things like "constructive criticism" become an oxymoron. If you are critical of an F from any standpoint, you can almost be certain they will be hurt. One of the biggest gifts the MBTI® offers, is the understanding of *why* we process certain things the way we do. For example, in this situation, the Feeler could learn that yes, it is okay to decide with your heart, but don't forget to balance it out by taking a step back and viewing the situation from the perspective of an observer. This is also helpful when dealing with Thinkers who may appear harsh or overly critical. Once it's understood that this is a decision making PROCESS, and not meant to be accusatory, these two preference types can come to much better understanding. (The same being true for the Thinker dealing with the Feeler: "Why do you take everything to heart?") In truth, as in all preference pairings, we can learn so much from one another.

J/P (Judging/Perceiving): *Our lifestyle...* Choosing **Perceiving** over Judging will usually result in being into open ends, spontaneity, and flexibility. (vs J closure, list making and structure). This could lead to a lot of unfinished projects as something gets started and the P is sidetracked by something 'more important.' The P probably doesn't get too ruffled when plans change and could even be known to change them just to shake things up a little. The natural leanings of the P could lead to viewing endless 'what ifs' when trying to come to closure, resulting in procrastination and not surprisingly, tardiness.

Incorporating a little of the the J's love of schedules could assist in being more organized. Once again the AWARENESS is invaluable. Many times we can be totally oblivious to certain personality characteristics until they are pointed out in tangible form. But remember, Type should never used as an excuse; for example, "It's okay for me to be involved in 12 different projects (and so who cares about completion), I'm a P." That's a no-go 'cause if you are aware of being a P, then you need to take the responsibility and work on the potential stumbling blocks associated with that preference. So there.

INFP, CHAKRAS & BALANCE

I will now acquaint you with suggested toolkits for the **INFP** that will include specific yoga postures, breathing practices (Pranayama) meditations, affirmations, and mudras (seals or 'hand yoga).

After an explanation of the 'toolkits' I have chosen to help enhance and maintain your natural strength as well as regain balance when necessary, there will be a short series of questions you can ask yourself to clarify just which energy field is most in need of attention.

Suggested Toolkits to Celebrate, Nurture & Restore Balance:
Heart Chakra, Solar Plexus Chakra, Root Chakra

(Depending on your particular life situation, ANY of the chakras may 'deserve' attention. You can determine this by reviewing the questions found in each toolkit.)

As a dominant Feeler (the "team captain" of your type) the heart chakra will be your home playing field. When life is flowing along in a healthy state, the **HEART CHAKRA TOOLKIT** is where you

106

can go to not only help maintain that balance, but to celebrate your gift of empathy, compassion and heart-based leadership.

This is also the flow you may choose to practice if you ask yourself the question, "Am I feeling depleted?" and the answer is 'yes.' This would be in cases of perhaps going through a period of grief or having given so much of yourself due to life circumstances that you find yourself needing a dose of heart chakra nourishment. This will allow you to open up both sides of the heart - able to give, but also able to receive and keep the energy circulating.

On the other hand if you are depleted due to an enabling situation, especially if you find yourself experiencing feelings of resentment, you will need to turn to your inferior function ("last to be asked to join the party"). In the case of the INFP, that refers to the Thinking Function and the **SOLAR PLEXUS TOOLKIT**. When the heart energy field is weakened or drained, we need to build up feelings of courage, confidence and self-esteem so that the playing field is leveled once again.

The INFP can be so filled with dreams and ideas that their feet no longer touch the ground. Combined with the element of Perceiving, this will also give rise to spending a bit of time in the clouds and a multitude of options. In the interest of reeling them into to the world of matter, spending time in **ROOT CHAKRA TOOLKIT** can bring you back to earth where the manifestation has a much better chance of taking place. Including a morning run or walk each day or just being out in nature and feeling your footfall on the earth also has a tremendously grounding influence.

All types need to be cognizant of the role that the throat chakra plays in our ability to communicate. The I-F will need to be wary of suppressing truth in the interest of not hurting anyone's feelings - at the expense of their own health and personal truth.

Questions for the INFP to ask themselves to determine which Chakra to nurture:

1) "Am I in a position where my heart is leading the way and I feel strong and giving?"

If YES, practice HEART CHAKRA TOOLKIT flows to maintain this sense of heart-felt leadership. If NO, due to depletion through grief or inability to receive the love you deserve, turn to this toolkit as well.

2) "Have I reached a point where I am sponge for other people's pain and feel unable to voice my frustration?"

If YES, practice **SOLAR PLEXUS CHAKRA** flows and meditations to increase the confidence and vigor within yourself. This 'fire' will reignite feelings of personal power that are necessary not only to enable you to practice self-care, but to continue to share love with others in your life from a healthy, balanced place.

3) Are you having a difficult time manifesting your heart dreams due to a myriad of options swirling around in your head?

If YES, turn to the ROOT CHAKRA TOOLKIT to reestabish your connection to the grounding of the earth element.

As always, no matter which energy field we are currently engaging, it is important to hold your intention in both mind and heart and then be open to the inspiration that follows.

ENERGY TYPES

INTP (Introverted-iNtuitive-Thinking-Perceiver) - Hellooooo In There!

*I*f the mind of the INTP was a mansion and you had the opportunity to explore all the rooms, I would suggest leaving breadcrumbs along your journey if you entertain any desire to find your way back out again! Intricate and analytical, this type, perhaps more than any other, has a burning desire to know *why* things work the way they do. And once they figure it out, they will probably have found an even better alternative to the status quo. As with most NT types (iNtuitive-Thinking), they are perfectionists and this expectation is not limited to their own endeavors, but to the world at large. If you ask for the opinion of the INTP, be prepared before anything else to hear, "Have you ever thought of doing it THIS way?" (Not that they don't appreciate your work thus far, but everything in their eyes is open to improvement.)

The team captain for the INTP is introverted Thinking and the wheels never stop spinning. What the world sees and hears are the endless possibilities behind these spinning wheels. Perchance. You may just see a person immersed in their own universe of ideas who, when spoken to, needs to be hailed back to the earth plane to join in the conversation. Add the P (Perceiving) to the equation and closure may be a pipe dream! (Here is another case where practicing a little structured J behavior definitely couldn't hurt.)

The INTP will tend to excel at whatever they put their mind to, due to those perfectionist tendencies as well as a quite competitive nature. Also typical of most NT types, they will be hardest on themselves if they have not lived up to their own level of expected competence.

They tend to see the world as one big puzzle that is begging to be deciphered. Because of this desire for knowledge, they are also inclined to be quite adventurous in the quest for quenching that thirst.

When under more than a 'healthy' amount of stress, the INTP could become quite melancholy and also start doing very uncharacteristic things like arranging their sock drawer. Now there's a red flag!

If you live with an INTP, it's quite easy to track them down because you can just follow the trail they leave upon arriving home. Hmmm.... jacket, shoes, wallet, keys, phone... a-ha! There you are! The physical world is but a landing place for much weightier issues to be examined.

From a relationship perspective, the INTP will probably be most content with a partner who is self-sufficient and allowing of their need for internalization and independence. They are quite dedicated once a commitment is made and from a daily life perspective, of importance to them will be just knowing you are there. There will be no real need for the bantering about of small talk. They will also wish for their family members the same level of peak life experiences that they themselves consider a natural part of life.

Careerwise, the INTP will be happiest when in a position that allows them freedom and room for experimentation. Structure is the bane of their world, unless they have created it. Even then, it will be ever evolving. Consequently, you will find the most content INTPs in areas such as scientific arenas (astronomy, etc), research and development, teaching at a university level, or possibly philosophy. One must also keep in mind that the strength of the INTP is most essentially in the creation and building phase of any undertaking because boredom will set in if they are expected to then be in charge of whatever it is they have devised.

Deep-thinking, competive and independent, the INTP introduces fresh (and often unexpected) new ways of perceiving our world.

HIERARCHY OF FUNCTION ("Who's On First?")

The middle two letters of a person's type - our 'functions' - will equate to how we experience (perceive) reality and how we make our decisions. The 'authority' as to which of these processes occurs first will vary by type. There is an order we go through when accessing them and this is pretty much determined by the 'comfort zones' of our individual type.

We each have...
a DOMINANT FUNCTION (Team Captain)
an AUXILIARY FUNCTION (Co-captain)
a TERTIARY FUNCTION (Third at bat)
and an INFERIOR FUNCTION (Benchwarmer)

Of note, the Extravert (E) will 'share' their dominant process with the world and internalize their auxiliary. The Introvert (I) will do the opposite, keeping their most preferred function internal and showing the world the 'next in command.'

This is the breakdown fo the INTP:
DOMINANT (introverted) T
AUXILIARY (extraverted) N
TERTIARY (introverted) S
INFERIOR (extraverted) F

Type Preference by Letter for the INTP:

E/I (Extraversion /Introversion): *How we are energized...* If you choose **Introversion** over Extraversion, you are usually most energized when spending quiet time alone or in the company of one or two close friends. You process things internally which Extraverts often find frustrating as they are not being kept up to date with minute by minute proceedings. If you want the most truthful, complete answer from an I, give them time to withdraw from the ruckus of the outer world and go within. Introverts also do not have the need to share their entire life story with people in line at the bank or sitting next to them on a plane. They are usually quite content to exist in their own universe until a need is felt to 'come out and play.' Now Introverts also need people, but being around too many people for too long a time can physically make them wither. As with all preferences, preservation of health means maintaining balance.

S/N (Sensing/iNtuition): *How we gather information...* This preference boils down to how we take in information, a vital component in communication. If we are experiencing *different* realities, learning to see things through the eyes of the receiving party will enable us to share in a way that will be understood. Choosing **iNtuition** over Sensing indicates being engaged in the world of possibilities, trusting gut feelings over past experience, looking to the future vs. what is currently 'on the table', and therefore not always being totally cognizant of what is going on right in front of one's nose. (e.g. walking right by something without seeing it if they aren't looking for it. And actually, sometimes even then). This is in contrast to the Sensor's comfort zone in the 'here and now' and trusting of five senses over conjecture.

114

T/F (Thinking/Feeling): *How we make our decisions...* These are both rational means of decision-making but one will almost always offer a much more natural approach. When **Thinking** is preferred over Feeling (again please recall that these are Jungian terms and don't indicate that we don't all do both) the decisions will be more from the head than the heart i.e. the T tends to take an objective stance apart from the situation vs becoming embedded in the process. While we all practice both modes of determination and one will be more natural, it is highly beneficial to learn to look at both sides of an issue, subjectively as well as objectively. In the world of the Feeler, this is where things like "constructive criticism" become an oxy-moron. If you are critical of an F from any standpoint, you can almost be certain they will be hurt. One of the biggest gifts the MBTI® offers, is the understanding of *why* we process certain things the way we do. For example, in this situation, the Feeler could learn that yes, it is okay to decide with your heart, but don't forget to bal-ance it out by taking a step back and viewing the situation from the perspective of an observer. This is also helpful when dealing with Thinkers who may appear harsh or overly critical. Once it's under-stood that this is a decision making PROCESS, and not meant to be accusatory, these two preference types can come to much better understanding. (The same being true for the Thinker dealing with the Feeler: "Why do you take everything to heart?") In truth, as in all preference pairings, we can learn so much from one another.

J/P (Judging/Perceiving): *Our lifestyle...* Choosing **Perceiving** over Judging will usually result in being into open ends, spontaneity, and flexibility. (vs J closure, list making and structure). This could lead to a lot of unfinished projects as something gets started and the P is sidetracked by something 'more important.' The P probably doesn't get too ruffled when plans change and could even be known to change them, just to shake things up a little. The natural leanings of the P could lead to viewing endless 'what ifs' when trying to come to closure, resulting in procrastination and not surprisingly, tardiness. Incorporating a little of the the J's love of schedules could assist in being more organized. Once again the AWARENESS is invaluable. Many times we can be totally oblivious to certain personality characteristics until they are pointed out in tangible form. But remember, Type should never used as an excuse; for example, "It's okay for me to be involved in 12 different projects (and so who cares about completion), I'm a P." That's a no-go 'cause if you are aware of being a P, then you need to take the responsibility and work on the potential stumbling blocks associated with that preference. So there.

INTP, CHAKRAS & BALANCE

I will now acquaint you with suggested toolkits for the **INTP** that will include specific yoga postures, breathing practices (Pranayama) meditations, affirmations, and mudras (seals or 'hand yoga).

After an explanation of the 'toolkits' I have chosen to help enhance and maintain your natural strength as well as regain balance when necessary, there will be a short series of questions you can ask yourself to clarify just which energy field is most in need of attention.

Suggested Toolkits to Celebrate, Nurture & Restore Balance:
Solar Plexus Chakra, Root Chakra, Heart Chakra

(Depending on your particular life situation, ANY of the chakras may 'deserve' attention. You can determine this by reviewing the questions found in each toolkit.)

The 'team captain' for the INTP, the Thinking function, will be a realm of natural strength. In order to celebrate this process, I would recommend practicing the flow and meditation found in the **SOLAR PLEXUS CHAKRA TOOLKIT**. Honoring this innate strength for analytical processing from a balanced state of confidence will enhance your ability to share it with the world. Should you feel depleted regarding the confidence necessary to move forward towards a goal, this is also a good place to start to rekindle the fire.

Taking your iNuitive co-captain into account coupled with your I (Introversion) and P (Perceiving) nature, you may have a strong tendency to spend gobs of time within that 'interior castle of options' ... so many possibilities, so many alternatives. If these ideas and plans are to come to fruition, engaging the **ROOT CHAKRA TOOLKIT** on a regular basis will offer the grounding necessary to usher them into manifestation.

As an iNtuitive Thinker (NT), you may need to spend some time getting in tune with the essence of what you are creating vs the perfection of the final outcome. Practicing the flow and meditation found within the **HEART CHAKRA TOOLKIT** should assist you in bringing clarity to what is truly most important. This field will also keep you in touch with the more subjective side within you (your 'benchwarmer' function') and allow you to be more cognizant and empathetic of the feelings of those sharing your life.

All types need to be cognizant of the role that the throat chakra plays in our ability to communicate. The I-T will need to be wary of avoiding issues because they feel 'uncomfortable' or 'none of my business.' But if areas of discomfort become suppressed rather than expressed, you may find that your health and emotional stability suffer as a result of not speaking your truth.

Questions for the INTP to ask themselves to determine which Chakra to nurture:

1) "Am I feeling confident and enthusiastic about sharing my ideas with the world?"

If YES, practice SOLAR PLEXUS flows and meditations with the intention of honoring your innate gifts of analysis and insight. If NO, then also turn to this toolkit to reinspire those strengths.

2) "Am I feeling slightly overwhelmed (or even completely untethered) as to how to harness the many ideas and desires swirling within my mind?"

If YES, practice ROOT CHAKRA flows and meditations to bring bring those inspirations and intentions back down to earth. (As mentioned above, the combo of Introversion, iNtuition and Perceiving invites routine visits to the Root Chakra Toolkit to help capitalize on the idea process.)

3) "Am I spending so much time in my own world that I am losing touch with the lives and feelings of those closest to me?"

If YES, practice HEART CHAKRA flows and meditations to reestablish loving contact with those who share your life, reinforcing what's truly most important. (Affirm that you are able to easily

accomplish your goals while still maintaining healthy relationships.)

*As always, no matter which energy field we are currently engaging, it is
important to hold your intention in both mind and heart and then be open
to the inspiration that follows.*

ENERGY TYPES

ESTP (Extraverted-Sensing-Thinking-Perceiver) - Life in the Fast Lane

*O*kay, picture a running track and all athletes lined up to burst forth into a 100 yard dash.... You are probably looking at a line up of ESTPs! (Well, maybe.) But that is the image that comes to mind when I think of this type. And I also can't help but think it's no coincidence that the last three letters are "STP," which also happen to designate engine oil, with Nascar/Richard Petty as the spokesperson. Go figure.

That being said, look for the ESTP to be involved in action-related pursuits that appeal to their dynamic way of life. As dominant Sensors (S), the first place they 'go' is into their world of perception which will include being very attentive to detail and their present surroundings. Next in line is the Thinking (T) process which they will visit to assist them in coming to logical conclusions. This will all be a quite verbal process considering their extraverted bent. Last but certainly not least, add to this their preference for a P lifestyle and you have the quintessential risk-taker. Life is made to be lived one second at a time!

As with most Sensing-Perceivers (SPs), any crisis situation will be handled with aplomb. It's just their nature to be on their toes regardless of the activity taking place around them. If things get TOO boring, they may even be known to throw some fuel on the fire to heat things up a bit.

121

With this description in mind, stress for the ESTP is probably the result of quite the opposite set of circumstances from most types. If things are stuck in 'status quo' with no end in sight, this will be the scenario that will cause this type to start feeling antsy and out of their comfort zone. Pacing, sighing, and generally out of sorts when life is 'on hold,' you may witness some very atypical behavior if there is no way out of this rut. This could include actually making deadlines and looking to the future for more possibilities to explore. (Unfortunately due to their troubled state of mind, however, their outlook could be quite negative regarding these options.)

The ESTP can achieve a very high standard in just about any endeavor, not out of the need for perfection, but rather from the sheer enjoyment of the pursuit that results in quality performance.

The ultimate realist, they are very in tune with their surroundings and their sense of recall of everything from a conversation they had with you last year to the color of their bedroom growing up will be just a thought away.

In an intimate relationship, it could take a while for them to even consider settling down. Commitment can be a scary thing for the ESTP. I mean, what if something better comes along? When they do finally agree to tie the knot, they will need space for their love of action and change. Their partner will have to be aware of this penchant for excitement if the relationship is to go 'long term.' (Remember, long term for the ESTP could mean more that a day or two.) If kids are part of the picture, they will most likely be brought up in a sporty, active environment.

In the world of work, the ESTP will be very motivated by an domain that offers change, action and attention to detail. News reporter, athlete, paramedic, stock broker or negotiation specialist are areas that come to mind that will keep the ESTP satisfied on the job.

Fun-loving, risk-taking realists, the ESTP adds verve and a dash of excitment to our world.

HIERARCHY OF FUNCTION ("Who's On First?")

The middle two letters of a person's type - our 'functions' - will equate to how we experience (perceive) reality and how we make our decisions. The 'authority' as to which of these processes occurs first will vary by type. There is an order we go through when accessing them and this is pretty much determined by the 'comfort zones' of our individual type.

We each have...
a DOMINANT FUNCTION (Team Captain)
an AUXILIARY FUNCTION (Co-captain)
a TERTIARY FUNCTION (Third at bat)
and an INFERIOR FUNCTION (Benchwarmer)

Of note, the Extravert (E) will 'share' their dominant process with the world and internalize their auxiliary. The Introvert (I) will do the opposite, keeping their most preferred function internal and showing the world the 'next in command.'

This is the breakdown fo the ESTP:
DOMINANT (extraverted) S
AUXILIARY (introverted) T
TERTIARY (extraverted) F
INFERIOR (introverted) N

Type Preference by Letter for the ESTP:

E/I (Extraversion /Introversion): *How we are energized...* If you choose **Extraversion** over Introversion, you are usually most energized when being in the company of others and sharing ideas. This does not mean that the E doesn't also require some quiet time. But having TOO much alone time for TOO long a period will be draining and the 'recharging process' will probably require some social interaction. Most Es will also talk their way through to making a point or coming to a decision as the entire thought process will be out in the open for all to hear. Now there exists a danger in this 'rambling' in that it could prove to be just that... rambling. Always confirm with an E exactly what you are hearing them say, especially if it involves YOU in any way just to make sure they aren't just venting aloud. The E may also have a hard time understanding why the I doesn't function in this same way and get frustrated when they need to play 'mind-reader.'

S/N (Sensing/iNtuition): *How we perceive reality...* This preference boils down to how take in information, a vital component in communication. If we are experiencing *different* realities, learning to see things through the eyes of the receiving party will enable us to share in a way that will be understood. If you choose **Sensing** over iNtuition, you are probably very engaged in the world of detail, the past and day-to-day experience. Living in the present and in the tactile world of the five senses - i.e. what you see, hear, taste, smell and touch - is your reality and you are quite attuned to your environment. (This in comparison to the iNtuitive who resides in the realm of possibilities, trusts 'gut feelings' over past experience, is future-oriented and not always cognizant of what is going on in the physical world. They tend to live beyond the 5 senses.) Being practical and dealing

with 'what is' as opposed to 'what could be' are key attributes of the Sensing Type. The S may also take things quite literally which the N should keep in mind when sharing information as miscommunication *could* run rampant. ("You SAID be here on the hour... but you DIDN'T say which one!") All in all, they can make great partners, but understanding the different modes of perception is essential.

T/F (Thinking/Feeling): *How we make our decisions...* These are both rational means of decision-making but one will almost always offer a much more natural approach. When **Thinking** is preferred over Feeling (again please recall that these are Jungian terms and don't indicate that we don't all do both) the decisions will be more from the head than the heart i.e. the T tends to take an objective stance apart from the situation vs becoming embedded in the process. While we all practice both modes of determination and one will be more natural, it is highly beneficial to learn to look at both sides of an issue, subjectively as well as objectively. In the world of the Feeler, this is where things like "constructive criticism" become an oxymoron. If you are critical of an F from any standpoint, you can almost be certain they will be hurt. One of the biggest gifts the MBTI® offers, is the understanding of *why* we process certain things the way we do. For example, in this situation, the Feeler could learn that yes, it is okay to decide with your heart, but don't forget to balance it out by taking a step back and viewing the situation from the perspective of an observer. This is also helpful when dealing with Thinkers who may appear harsh or overly critical. Once it's understood that this is a decision making PROCESS, and not meant to be accusatory, these two preference types can come to much better understanding. (The same being true for the Thinker dealing with the Feeler: "Why do you take everything to heart?") In truth, as in all preference pairings, we can learn so much from one another.

J/P (Judging/Perceiving): *Our lifestyle...* Choosing **Perceiving** over Judging will usually result in being into open ends, spontaneity, and flexibility. (vs J closure, list making and structure). This could lead to a lot of unfinished project as something gets started and the P is sidetracked by something 'more important.' The P probably doesn't get too ruffled when plans change and could even be known to change them, just to shake things up a little. The natural leanings of the P could lead to viewing endless 'what ifs' when trying to come to closure, resulting in procrastination and not surprisingly, tardiness. Incorporating a little of the the J's love of schedules could assist in being more organized. Once again the AWARENESS is invaluable. Many times we can be totally oblivious to certain personality characteristics until they are pointed out in tangible form. But remember, Type should never used as an excuse; for example, "It's okay for me to be involved in 12 different projects (and so who cares about completion), I'm a P." That's a no-go 'cause if you are aware of being a P, then you need to take the responsibility and work on the potential stumbling blocks associated with that preference. So there.

ESTP, CHAKRAS & BALANCE

I will now acquaint you with suggested toolkits for the **ESTP** that will include specific yoga postures, breathing practices (Pranayama) meditations, affirmations, and mudras (seals or 'hand yoga).

After an explanation of the 'toolkits' I have chosen to help enhance and maintain your natural strength as well as regain balance when necessary, there will be a short series of questions you can ask yourself to clarify just which energy field is most in need of attention.

Suggested Toolkits to Celebrate, Nurture & Restore Balance:
Sacral Chakra, Root Chakra, Heart Chakra

(Depending on your particular life situation, ANY of the chakras may 'deserve' attention. You can determine this by reviewing the questions found in each toolkit.)

The combination of being a dominant Sensor ("team captain" of your type) along with a P lifestyle, (S-P) results in a flexible, spontaneous personality type. You are at your best when embracing the unpredictable and you shine when you are able to put your love of action into concrete results. To keep the motivation rolling, the **SACRAL CHAKRA TOOLKIT** will enhance your natural born gifts. This is also the place to turn if you feel that your momentum is slacking as this energy field is all about flow, movement and the water element. This will augment the desire to create, to remain flexible and also increase tolerance in relationships.

Maintaining a balanced **ROOT CHAKRA** is also important, because your love of change and action can sometimes play havoc with your ability to commit or come to closure. This toolkit will enable you to incorporate the structure you may need to stay grounded and stable.

As you typically experience your comfort zone when living in the moment and searching out the 'next big wave,' you could find that your heart chakra is not getting the attention it needs. This could occur from two different perspectives: Allowing yourself to accept and appreciate the love and attention being offered you or in your ability to share love, compassion and appreciation with the others in your life. Spending time in the **HEART CHAKRA TOOLKIT** can offer you the balance that will keep the relationship with yourself as well others in a healthy state.

All types need to be cognizant of the role that the throat chakra plays in our ability to communicate. The E-T will need to be wary of blurting out an opinion that may not actually be representative of what they are really feeling at all. But once it's out there, it's hard to take it back and the damage could already be done.

Questions for the ESTP to ask themselves to determine which Chakra to nurture:

1) "Am I feeling enthusiastic and motivated to explore and enhance my life path?"

If YES, practice SACRAL CHAKRA flows and meditations with the intention of riding the flow of creativity and expansion. If NO, practice SACRAL CHAKRA toolkit offerings to help bring you back into your natural spontaneous life gifts.

2) "Am I feeling unable to make commitments or bring about necessary closure that will bring structure to my life plans?"

If YES, practice ROOT CHAKRA flows and meditations to connect you to the earth element of rootedness and stability. Allow that fertile ground to be a foundation for the seeds of your creativity.

3) "Do I feel blocked when it comes to giving and receiving love and affection in my life?"

If YES, practice HEART CHAKRA flows and meditations to increase your ability to be open to self-love and care as well as the warmth that others in your life desire to share with you.

As always, no matter which energy field we are currently engaging, it is important to hold your intention in both mind and heart and then be open to the inspiration that follows.

ENERGY TYPES

ESFP (Extraverted-Sensing-Feeling-Perceiver) - Here To Enjoy the Ride

*I*f any type was born with rose-colored glasses, it would be the ESFP, but auspiciously I must add. Life is meant to be lived to the fullest, every moment of every day as they choose to see the glass as half full. As dominant Sensors (S), their world is a fascinating, ever-changing array of experiences to take part in. Add to this their Perceiving (P) nature and these undertakings will most certainly not be governed by a clock or a calendar (if that can be avoided.) The options for exploring are endless and this is definitely another type scenario where boredom does not fit into their vocabulary.

The co-captain for this type is Feeling and not always readily visible to the world. But while adventure is high on the agenda, altruism will enter the picture as they turn the focus inward to consider the feelings of others in their lives.

The combo of Sensing and Perceiving (S-P) will sometimes effect their ability to come to closure as they are more interested in gathering information and testing alternatives than in making a commitment. This also adds to their sense of adaptability should plans change midstream. "Hey, go with the flow!" will be the most likely response to situations where other types would be going grey. This versatility can also make the ESFP quite capable in emergency situations.

Their attraction to a steady diet of stimulation can also lead to a schedule that is brimming over as they attempt to take on more and more activities. It is not out of the ordinary for an ESFP to hit the gym prior to work, have a different lunch date every day during break time, attend a class in the evening to learn some new skill and then cap the evening off with a movie and popcorn. Where DO they get the energy?

Now when the ESFP undergoes a higher than normal amount of stress, you may not recognize them whatsoever. This is especially true if their sense of ethics is being threatened. It's out the window with the devil-may-care attitude only to be replaced by the iron will of a warrior. The penchant for detail will become a passion for exploring every possibility and the easy-going P will begin to demand closure around each of these alternatives. This may also lead to a tendency to expect the worst...until the waters have calmed again.

While typically a fan of the romantic, the ESFP in an intimate relationship will probably choose to express this in a nontraditional manner. Treasure hunts through flea markets to find a birthday gift , hot air ballooning with a bottle of champagne under a full moon, hiring a singing tomato to surprise you in your office on your aniversary... in other words, if adventure speaks to you, you're in. If not, it may be best to seek out a more subdued companion. The children of the ESFP will be encouraged to try new and different activities as well, not with the aim of perfection in mind, but just for the sake of experiencing the unfamiliar and exotic.

From a career standpoint, the ESFP can excel in a number of areas, but will probably be happiest when able to work in a social atmosphere that calls for innovative input and minimal structure. Areas they could excel in run the gamut of retail sales to real estate to paramedics. If the atmosphere calls for same 'ol, same 'ol, then the boredom will set in and they will be off to greener pastures. While earning a living is important, the achievement of inner gratification is of most significance.

Gregarious, fun-loving, and quick on the uptake, the ESFP adds more than their fair share of joy to our world.

HIERARCHY OF FUNCTION ("Who's On First?")

The middle two letters of a person's type - our 'functions' - will equate to how we experience (perceive) reality and how we make our decisions. The 'authority' as to which of these processes occurs first will vary by type. There is an order we go through when accessing them and this is pretty much determined by the 'comfort zones' of our individual type.

We each have...
a DOMINANT FUNCTION (Team Captain)
an AUXILIARY FUNCTION (Co-captain)
a TERTIARY FUNCTION (Third at bat)
and an INFERIOR FUNCTION (Benchwarmer)

Of note, the Extravert (E) will 'share' their dominant process with the world and internalize their auxiliary. The Introvert (I) will do the opposite, keeping their most preferred function internal and showing the world the 'next in command.'

This is the breakdown fo the ESFP:
DOMINANT (extraverted) S
AUXILIARY (introverted) F
TERTIARY (extraverted) T
INFERIOR (introverted) N

Type Preference by Letter for the ESFP:

E/I (Extraversion /Introversion): *How we are energized...* If you choose **Extraversion** over Introversion, you are usually most energized when being in the company of others and sharing ideas. This does not mean that the E doesn't also require some quiet time. But having TOO much alone time for TOO long a period will be draining and the 'recharging process' will probably require some social interaction. Most Es will also talk their way through to making a point or coming to a decision as the entire thought process will be out in the open for all to hear. Now there exists a danger in this 'rambling' in that it could prove to be just that... rambling. Always confirm with an E exactly what you are hearing them say, especially if it involves YOU in any way just to make sure they aren't just venting aloud. The E may also have a hard time understanding why the I doesn't function in this same way and get frustrated when they need to play 'mind-reader.'

S/N (Sensing/iNtuition): *How we perceive reality...* This preference boils down to how take in information, a vital component in communication. If we are experiencing *different* realities, learning to see things through the eyes of the receiving party will enable us to share in a way that will be understood. If you choose **Sensing** over iNtuition, you are probably very engaged in the world of detail, the past and day-to-day experience. Living in the present and in the tactile world of the five senses - i.e. what you see, hear, taste, smell and touch - is your reality and you are quite attuned to your environment. (This in comparison to the iNtuitive who resides in the realm of possibilities, trusts 'gut feelings' over past experience, is future-oriented and not always cognizant of what is going on in the physical world. They tend to live beyond the 5 senses.) Being practical and dealing

with 'what is' as opposed to 'what could be' are key attributes of the Sensing Type. The S may also take things quite literally which the N should keep in mind when sharing information as miscommunication *could* run rampant. ("You SAID be here on the hour... but you DIDN'T say which one!") All in all, they can make great partners, but understanding the different modes of perception is essential.

T/F (Thinking/Feeling): *How we make our decisions...* If you choose **Feeling** over Thinking as your method of decision making, you tend to become embedded in the situation you are currently encountering. While we all practice both modes of determination, this arena will most often be a more comfortable fit for you. And though one will feel more natural, it is highly beneficial to learn to look at both sides of an issue, subjectively as well as objectively. In the world of the Feeler, this is where things like "constructive criticism" become an oxymoron. If you are critical of an F from any standpoint, you can almost be certain they will be hurt. One of the biggest gifts the MBTI® offers, is the understanding of *why* we process certain things the way we do. For example, in this situation, the Feeler could learn that yes, it is okay to decide with your heart, but don't forget to balance it out by taking a step back and viewing the situation from the perspective of an observer. This is also helpful when dealing with Thinkers who may appear harsh or overly critical. Once it's understood that this is a decision making PROCESS, and not meant to be accusatory, these two preference types can come to much better understanding. (The same being true for the Thinker dealing with the Feeler: "Why do you take everything to heart?") In truth, as in all preference pairings, we can learn so much from one another.

J/P (Judging/Perceiving): *Our lifestyle...* Choosing **Perceiving** over Judging will usually result in being into open ends, spontaneity, and flexibility. (vs J closure, list making and structure). This could lead to a lot of unfinished projects as something gets started and the P is sidetracked by something 'more important.' The P probably doesn't get too ruffled when plans change and could even be known to change them, just to shake things up a little. The natural leanings of the P could lead to viewing endless 'what ifs' when trying to come to closure, resulting in procrastination and not surprisingly, tardiness. Incorporating a little of the the J's love of schedules could assist in being more organized. Once again the AWARENESS is invaluable. Many times we can be totally oblivious to certain personality characteristics until they are pointed out in tangible form. But remember, Type should never used as an excuse; for example, "It's okay for me to be involved in 12 different projects (and so who cares about completion), I'm a P." That's a no-go 'cause if you are aware of being a P, then you need to take the responsibility and work on the potential stumbling blocks associated with that preference. So there.

ESFP, CHAKRAS & BALANCE

I will now acquaint you with suggested toolkits for the **ESFP** that will include specific yoga postures, breathing practices (Pranayama) meditations, affirmations, and mudras (seals or 'hand yoga).

After an explanation of the 'toolkits' I have chosen to help enhance and maintain your natural strength as well as regain balance when necessary, there will be a short series of questions you can ask yourself to clarify just which energy field is most in need of attention.

Suggested Toolkits to Celebrate, Nurture & Restore Balance:
Sacral Chakra, Root Chakra, Third Eye Chakra

(Depending on your particular life situation, ANY of the chakras may 'deserve' attention. You can determine this by reviewing the questions found in each toolkit.)

The combination of being a dominant Sensor ("team captain" of your type) along with a P lifestyle, (S-P) results in a flexible, spontaneous personality type. You are at your best when embracing the unpredictable and you shine when you are able to step up to the plate with new and exciting ideas. To keep the motivation rolling, the **SACRAL CHAKRA TOOLKIT** will enhance your natural born gifts. This is also the place to turn if you feel that your momentum is slacking as this energy field is all about flow, movement and the water element. This will augment the desire to create as well as increase tolerance in relationships.

Maintaining a balanced **ROOT CHAKRA** is also important, because your love of change and action can sometimes play havoc with your ability to commit or come to closure. This toolkit will enable you incorporate the structure you may need to stay grounded and stable.

As you typically experience your comfort zone when living in the moment, you may also find spending time in the **THIRD EYE CHAKRA TOOLKIT** to be beneficial. Embrace this internal realm, especially if you are in the middle of any situation that demands relying on your intuition. 'Ajna' will remove you from the hectic demands of the every day and allow you to turn inward to access the wisdom of your inner vision.

All types need to be cognizant of the role that the throat chakra plays in our ability to communicate. The E-F will need to be wary of either suppressing truth in the interest of not hurting anyone's feelings or sugar coating a situation that is in need of honest communication. This is at the expense of their own health and personal truth.

Questions for the ESFP to ask themselves to determine which Chakra to nurture:

1) *"Am I feeling enthusiastic and motivated to explore and enhance my life path?"*

If YES, practice SACRAL CHAKRA flows and meditations with the intention of riding the flow of creativity and expansion. If NO, practice SACRAL CHAKRA toolkit offerings to help bring you back into your natural spontaneous life gifts.

2) *"Am I feeling unable to make commitments or bring about necessary closure that will bring structure to my life plans?"*

If YES, practice ROOT CHAKRA flows and meditations to connect you to the earth element of rootedness and stability. Allow that fertile ground to be a foundation for the seeds of your creativity.

3) *"Do I sense a need to explore beyond the daily list of to-dos and access a deeper sense of inner vision?"*

If YES, practice THIRD EYE CHAKRA flows and meditations to embrace the innate sense of intuition that is available to us all when we bring our focus inward. Turn off the static of the outside world as you affirm the guidance that will come when you access this place of knowing.

As always, no matter which energy field we are currently engaging, it is important to hold your intention in both mind and heart and then be open to the inspiration that follows.

ENERGY TYPES

ENFP (Extraverted-Intuitive-Feeling-Perceiver)
- Dream Every Dream...

$\mathcal{O}$f perhaps all of the sixteen types, the ENFP has a particular knack for getting the ball rolling whether it's an event at work or a fundraiser for a close-to-the-heart cause. They will have a plethora of ideas on how it should all play out, with iNtuition being their 'team captain' and this means that the possibilities are endless. Now pair that up with their P and while they indeed have many wonderful suggestions to share, it would be advisable to have a J standing in the wings to make sure things transpire on time or all that energy can go up in smoke. (But boy can they throw a party!)

The social calendar of the ENFP is notoriously full. If you wish to spend time with them, book early... but be sure to remind them prior to the date or they may recall your rendez-vous a week later. Typically quite gregarious, the ENFP will have friends and acquaintances from a variety of backgrounds and take great pleasure in their ever-expanding circle of 'family.' The word boredom has no place in their vocabulary because the world to them is truly a banquet to be savored, a delicacy here, a delicacy there. But some may occasionally question whether there is a concrete direction behind all this activity and the ENFP readily knows the answer to that. Of *course* there is. They would, though, be wise to keep in mind that building castles in the air is indeed a trait of many N-Ps. Inviting some closure-oriented elements into their lifestyle will help assure that the foundation is built beneath them and then watch the process evolve beautifully.

When dealing with the ENFP, the world hears all about options and prospects, but what's going on underneath the surface is the F trying to figure out how all these plans are going to affect and/or help people.

If you hurt the feelings of an ENFP, it will usually become promptly apparent because their natural verve could be overtaken by an aloofness that you may not have even known existed. Under stress, a tendency exists to 'communicate' with language that could cut to the quick after which they may sequester themselves in an atypical island of rigidity.

In a relationship, they will see an abundance of directions that the alliance could take. They may also initially look beyond what at first appears an incompatible characteristic if they can envision the potential behind it. This, of course, can be a blessing as well as a curse, given that going into a relationship in the hopes of changing someone, no matter how much you believe in them, can backfire. In any case, romance, intrigue and creative avenues of sharing will all be a defininte enticement to this type.

Careerwise, their slogan could be, "Don't fence me in!" As with the aforementioned banquet table, they are most satisfied when able to dabble in a number of different areas, putting their many talents to use. Most often (happily) found in positions that take advantage of their social skills, they would likely find satisfaction in service industries surrounding arts, food, music or hospitality. Acting could also be a big draw as well as psychology or retail sales (of a product for which they have a personal fondness).

Enthusiastic, outgoing and perceptive, the ENFP offers the world a unique zest for life.

HIERARCHY OF FUNCTION ("Who's On First?")

The middle two letters of a person's type - our 'functions' - will equate to how we experience (perceive) reality and how we make our decisions. The 'authority' as to which of these processes occurs first will vary by type. There is an order we go through when accessing them and this is pretty much determined by the 'comfort zones' of our individual type.

We each have...
a DOMINANT FUNCTION (Team Captain)
an AUXILIARY FUNCTION (Co-captain)
a TERTIARY FUNCTION (Third at bat)
and an INFERIOR FUNCTION (Benchwarmer)

Of note, the Extravert (E) will 'share' their dominant process with the world and internalize their auxiliary. The Introvert (I) will do the opposite, keeping their most preferred function internal and showing the world the 'next in command.'

This is the breakdown fo the ENFP:
DOMINANT (extraverted) N
AUXILIARY (introverted) F
TERTIARY (extraverted) T
INFERIOR (introverted) S

Type Preference by Letter for the ENFP:

E/I (Extraversion /Introversion): *How we are energized...* If you choose **Extraversion** over Introversion, you are usually most energized when being in the company of others and sharing ideas. This does not mean that the E doesn't also require some quiet time. But having TOO much alone time for TOO long a period will be draining and the 'recharging process' will probably require some social interaction. Most Es will also talk their way through to making a point or coming to a decision as the entire thought process will be out in the open for all to hear. Now there exists a danger in this 'rambling' in that it could prove to be just that... rambling. Always confirm with an E exactly what you are hearing them say, especially if it involves YOU in any way just to make sure they aren't just venting aloud. The E may also have a hard time understanding why the I doesn't function in this same way and get frustrated when they need to play 'mind-reader.'

S/N (Sensing/iNtuition): *How we gather information...* This preference boils down to how we take in information, a vital component in communication. If we are experiencing *different* realities, learning to see things through the eyes of the receiving party will enable us to share in a way that will be understood. Choosing **iNtuition** over Sensing indicates being engaged in the world of possibilities, trusting gut feelings over past experience, looking to the future vs. what is currently 'on the table', and therefore not always being totally cognizant of what is going on right in front of one's nose. (e.g. walking right by something without seeing it if they aren't looking for it. And actually, sometimes even then). This is in contrast to the Sensor's comfort zone in the 'here and now' and trusting of five senses over conjecture.

T/F (Thinking/Feeling): *How we make our decisions...* If you choose **Feeling** over Thinking as your method of decision making, you tend to become embedded in the situation you are currently encountering. While we all practice both modes of determination, this arena will most often be a more comfortable fit for you. And though one will feel more natural, it is highly beneficial to learn to look at both sides of an issue, subjectively as well as objectively. In the world of the Feeler, this is where things like "constructive criticism" become an oxymoron. If you are critical of an F from any standpoint, you can almost be certain they will be hurt. One of the biggest gifts the MBTI® offers, is the understanding of *why* we process certain things the way we do. For example, in this situation, the Feeler could learn that yes, it is okay to decide with your heart, but don't forget to balance it out by taking a step back and viewing the situation from the perspective of an observer. This is also helpful when dealing with Thinkers who may appear harsh or overly critical. Once it's understood that this is a decision making PROCESS, and not meant to be accusatory, these two preference types can come to much better understanding. (The same being true for the Thinker dealing with the Feeler: "Why do you take everything to heart?") In truth, as in all preference pairings, we can learn so much from one another.

J/P (Judging/Perceiving): *Our lifestyle...* Choosing **Perceiving** over Judging will usually result in being into open ends, spontaneity, and flexibility. (vs J closure, list making and structure). This could lead to a lot of unfinished project as something gets started and the P is sidetracked by something 'more important.' The P probably doesn't get too ruffled when plans change and could even be known to change them, just to shake things up a little. The natural leanings of the P could lead to viewing endless 'what ifs' when trying to come to

closure, resulting in procrastination and not surprisingly, tardiness..
Incorporating a little of the the J's love of schedules could assist in
being more organized. Once again the AWARENESS is invaluable.
Many times we can be totally oblivious to certain personality characteristics until they are pointed out in tangible form. But remember,
Type should never be used as an excuse; for example, "It's okay for
me to be involved in 12 different projects (and so who cares about
completion), I'm a P." That's a no-go 'cause if you are aware of being
a P, then you need to take the responsibility and work on the potential stumbling blocks associated with that preference. So there.

ENFP, CHAKRAS & BALANCE

I will now acquaint you with suggested toolkits for the **ENFP** that
will include specific yoga postures, breathing practices (Pranayama)
meditations, affirmations, and mudras (seals or 'hand yoga).

After an explanation of the 'toolkits' I have chosen to help enhance
and maintain your natural strength as well as regain balance when
necessary, there will be a short series of questions you can ask yourself to clarify just which energy field is most in need of attention.

Suggested Toolkits to Celebrate, Nurture & Restore Balance:
Third Eye Chakra, Root Chakra, Heart Chakra

*(Depending on your particular life situation, ANY of the chakras may 'deserve' attention.
You can determine this by reviewing the questions found in each toolkit.)*

The 'team captain' for the ENFP, the iNtuitive perceiving function
will be a realm of natural strength. In order to celebrate this process,
I would recommend practicing the flow and meditation found in the

THIRD EYE CHAKRA TOOLKIT. Especially if you find yourself at a time in your life where dreams and 'gut feelings' are particulary strong and accurate, this will help bring even further clarity to your path.

Now, it is important to recognize the tendency for a dominant N to also spend an inordinate amount of time in that 'interior castle of options.' In order to allow these ideas to blossom into more than just passing fancies, combining Third Eye Chakra flow with the tools found within the **ROOT CHAKRA TOOLKIT** would give foundation to these dreams through the incorporation of stablity and grounding. Including a morning run or walk each day or just being out in nature and feeling your footfall on the earth also has a tremendously grounding influence.

The **THIRD EYE CHAKRA TOOLKIT** will also be of benefit should you feel yourself UNABLE to access that normal myriad of ideas. You can 'rev it up' through a similar process, just focusing on a different intention. ("I now open myself to new and beautiful inspirational ideas.")

Your 'co-captain,' the Feeling function, will also prove key in supporting these visions by bringing you into a decision-making mode. As an iNtuitive Feeler (NF) there may be the propensity for overextending yourself in the realm of rescuing. Narrowing the plethora of possibilities down to a manageable, concrete plan will streamline your intent. Practicing the flow and meditation found within the **HEART CHAKRA TOOLKIT** should assist you in bringing clarity to what is truly most important.

147

All types need to be cognizant of the role that the throat chakra plays in our ability to communicate. The E-F will need to be wary of either suppressing truth in the interest of not hurting anyone's feelings or sugar coating a situation that is in need of honest communication. This is at the expense of their own health and personal truth.

Questions for the ENFP to ask themselves to determine which Chakra to nurture:

1) "Am I feeling energized and productive in relation to the beautiful possibilities in my life?"

If YES, practice THIRD EYE CHAKRA flows and meditations with the intention of honoring your innate gifts of 'seeing' the vast playing field of options and alternatives. If NO, then also turn to this toolkit to reinspire those strengths.

2) "Am I feeling slightly overwhelmed (or even completely untethered) as to how to harness the many ideas and desires swirling within my mind?"

If YES, practice ROOT CHAKRA flows and meditations to bring bring those inspirations and intentions back down to earth. (As mentioned above, the combo of Third Eye and Root Chakra is pretty much always recommended to capitalize on the idea process.)

3) "Am I longing to put my project into action but experiencing a sense of confusion concerning who I can assist and how?" And/or, "Do I feel comfort in giving but have a difficult time receiving the same offers of generosity?"

If YES, practice HEART CHAKRA flows and meditations to bring yourself into an authentic place within your own heart where a knowing will unfold and establish a framework for manifestation. (Affirm that you are centered and focused in targeting your vision.)

As always, no matter which energy field we are currently engaging, it is important to hold your intention in both mind and heart and then be open to the inspiration that follows.

ENERGY TYPES

ENTP (Extraverted-iNtuitive-Thinking-Perceiver) - Look Out World, Here I Come!

*D*o you know that feeling when a storm is approaching but you aren't quite sure when and where it will hit? Well, the ENTP can create similar vibes when they enter a room. What was generally quiet and stable could turn topsy-turvy when the energy of this type shows up on the scene! Ideas will flow at lightning speed and before you have been able to digest *one* of these concepts, they will be on to a completely different set of visions because the last one was already becoming passé. The dominant iNtuitive process of the ENTP is an extraverted one and thus, those in proximity get showered in their fount of limitless possibilities.

The enthusiasm this type generates leads them into a variety of activities in their personal world as well as the work arena. As with most NTs (iNtuitive Thinkers) their standards are extremely high and this need for perfection can be both a gift as well as a curse. Being motivated by a benchmark that defies logic can set the ENTP up for disappointment if the caliber of their work does not live up to their own expectations. Add to this the likelihood that they will be bored with the process long before completion and you have a double whammy in the satisfaction department. This is usually due to the fact that this type is much more energized by the pursuit of an idea rather than the consummation...

This talent for postulating makes the ENTP probably the most likely to succeed in the arena of entrepreneurship. The combination of being 'big picture" people as well as loving to generate alternatives sets the stage for futuristic ventures.

They have a natural tendency for playing devil's advocate just because it's 'fun' to challenge others to see the opposing side of an issue. Now, those 'others' may not be quite as into the game as the ENTP, so it might behoove this type to test the waters before saying "en garde."

Under stress, you could first witness a defensiveness, almost as if a coat of armor is being suited in anticipation of a battle. If the stress intensifies, a very atypical wall of silence might arise, behind which the ENTP may withdraw into a melancholy state.

From a relationship standpoint, the ENTP can be boldly romantic, for example, arriving on a white stallion bearing a dozen gold roses. The person entering a partnership with this type would best be adventurous, flexible and ready to push the limits. (Having a liking for closure might also be a good idea, though not necessarily one that will be appreciated by the ENTP. This would be more for the general health of the relationship.) 'Pairing up' with this go-getter will definitely be stimulating, but could also prove a bit exhausting! If children enter the picture, you can be sure that the ENTP will see to it that they have all the latest gadgets as well as opportunities to excel in a variety of extracurricular activities.

In the career domain, again look for entrepreneurial leanings that could manifest in a variety of settings. Give them the space they need if you want them to express their most natural, God-given talents.

Areas that may be of strongest interest could be technology, sales, cutting edge legal work, or in the speaker arena.

For the ENTP, the world is their stage and the play is ever-changing and expanding.

HIERARCHY OF FUNCTION ("Who's On First?")

The middle two letters of a person's type - our 'functions' - will equate to how we experience (perceive) reality and how we make our decisions. The 'authority' as to which of these processes occurs first will vary by type. There is an order we go through when accessing them and this is pretty much determined by the 'comfort zones' of our individual type.

We each have...
a DOMINANT FUNCTION (Team Captain)
an AUXILIARY FUNCTION (Co-captain)
a TERTIARY FUNCTION (Third at bat)
and an INFERIOR FUNCTION (Benchwarmer)

Of note, the Extravert (E) will 'share' their dominant process with the world and internalize their auxiliary. The Introvert (I) will do the opposite, keeping their most preferred function internal and showing the world the 'next in command.'

This is the breakdown fo the ENTP:
DOMINANT (extraverted) N
AUXILIARY (introverted) T
TERTIARY (extraverted) F
INFERIOR (introverted) S

Type Preference by Letter for the ENTP:

E/I (Extraversion /Introversion): *How we are energized...* If you choose **Extraversion** over Introversion, you are usually most energized when being in the company of others and sharing ideas. This does not mean that the E doesn't also require some quiet time. But having TOO much alone time for TOO long a period will be draining and the 'recharging process' will probably require some social interaction. Most Es will also talk their way through to making a point or coming to a decision as the entire thought process will be out in the open for all to hear. Now there exists a danger in this 'rambling' in that it could prove to be just that... rambling. Always confirm with an E exactly what you are hearing them say, especially if it involves YOU in any way just to make sure they aren't just venting aloud. The E may also have a hard time understanding why the I doesn't function in this same way and get frustrated when they need to play 'mind-reader.'

S/N (Sensing/iNtuition): *How we gather information...* This preference boils down to how we take in information, a vital component in communication. If we are experiencing *different* realities, learning to see things through the eyes of the receiving party will enable us to share in a way that will be understood. Choosing **iNtuition** over Sensing indicates being engaged in the world of possibilities, trusting gut feelings over past experience, looking to the future vs. what is currently 'on the table', and therefore not always being totally cognizant of what is going on right in front of one's nose. (e.g. walking right by something without seeing it if they aren't looking for it. And actually, sometimes even then). This is in contrast to the Sensor's comfort zone in the 'here and now' and trusting of five senses over conjecture.

T/F (Thinking/Feeling): *How we make our decisions...* These are both rational means of decision-making but one will almost always offer a much more natural approach. When **Thinking** is preferred over Feeling (again please recall that these are Jungian terms and don't indicate that we don't all do both) the decisions will be more from the head than the heart i.e. the T tends to take an objective stance apart from the situation vs becoming embedded in the process. While we all practice both modes of determination and one will be more natural, it is highly beneficial to learn to look at both sides of an issue, subjectively as well as objectively. In the world of the Feeler, this is where things like "constructive criticism" become an oxymoron. If you are critical of an F from any standpoint, you can almost be certain they will be hurt. One of the biggest gifts the MBTI® offers, is the understanding of *why* we process certain things the way we do. For example, in this situation, the Feeler could learn that yes, it is okay to decide with your heart, but don't forget to balance it out by taking a step back and viewing the situation from the perspective of an observer. This is also helpful when dealing with Thinkers who may appear harsh or overly critical. Once it's understood that this is a decision making PROCESS, and not meant to be accusatory, these two preference types can come to much better understanding. (The same being true for the Thinker dealing with the Feeler: "Why do you take everything to heart?") In truth, as in all preference pairings, we can learn so much from one another.

J/P (Judging/Perceiving): *Our lifestyle...* Choosing **Perceiving** over Judging will usually result in being into open ends, spontaneity, and flexibility. (vs J closure, list making and structure). This could lead to a lot of unfinished projects as something gets started and the P is sidetracked by something 'more important.' The P probably doesn't get too ruffled when plans change and could even be known to just to shake things up a little. The natural leanings of the P could lead to viewing endless 'what ifs' when trying to come to closure. Procrastination and being on time could be the result of this. Incorporating a little of the the J's love of schedules could assist in being more organized. Once again the AWARENESS is invaluable. Many times we can be totally oblivious to certain personality characteristics until they are pointed out in tangible form. But remember, Type should never used as an excuse; for example, "It's okay for me to be involved in 12 different projects (and so who cares about completion), I'm a P." That's a no-go 'cause if you are aware of being a P, then you need to take the responsibility and work on the potential stumbling blocks associated with that preference. So there.

ENTP, CHAKRAS & BALANCE

I will now acquaint you with suggested toolkits for the **ENTP** that will include specific yoga postures, breathing practices (Pranayama) meditations, affirmations, and mudras (seals or 'hand yoga).

After an explanation of the 'toolkits' I have chosen to help enhance and maintain your natural strength as well as regain balance when necessary, there will be a short series of questions you can ask yourself to clarify just which energy field is most in need of attention.

Suggested Toolkits to Celebrate, Nurture & Restore Balance:
Third Eye Chakra, Root Chakra, Heart Chakra
(Depending on your particular life situation, ANY of the chakras may 'deserve' attention. You can determine this by reviewing the questions found in each toolkit.)

The 'team captain' for the ENTP, dominant iNtuition, will be a realm of natural strength. In order to celebrate this process, I would recommend practicing the flow and meditation found in the **THIRD EYE CHAKRA TOOLKIT.** Especially if you find yourself at a time in your life where dreams and 'gut feelings' are particulary strong and accurate, this will help bring even further clarity to your path.

Now, it is important to recognize the tendency for a dominant N to also spend an inordinate amount of time in the realm of possibilities. Add to this the plethora of options that your P (Perceiving) nature gladly bestows upon you and it will become imperative to access some grounding energy if you desire that your ideas become more than just passing fancies. So, combining Third Eye Chakra flow with the tools found within the **ROOT CHAKRA TOOLKIT** can give foundation to these dreams by accessing the stability necessary for their manifestation.

The **THIRD EYE CHAKRA TOOLKIT** will also be of benefit should you feel yourself UNABLE to access that normal myriad of ideas. You can 'rev it up' through a similar process, just focusing on a different intention. ("I now open myself to new and beautiful inspirational ideas.")

Your 'co-captain', the Thinking function, will also prove key in supporting these visions by bringing you into a decision-making mode. As an iNtuitive Thinker (NT), though, you may need to spend some time getting in tune with the essence of what you are creating vs the perfection of the final outcome. Practicing the flow and meditation found within the **HEART CHAKRA TOOLKIT** should assist you in bringing clarity to what is truly most important.

All types need to be cognizant of the role that the throat chakra plays in our ability to communicate. The E-T will need to be wary of blurting out an opinion that may not actually be representative of what they are really feeling at all. But once it's out there, it's hard to take it back and the damage could already be done.

Questions for the ENTP to ask themselves to determine which Chakra to nurture:

1) "Am I feeling energized and productive in relation to the beautiful possibilities in my life?"

If YES, practice **THIRD EYE CHAKRA** flows and meditations with the intention of honoring your innate gifts of 'seeing' the vast playing field of options and alternatives. If NO, then also turn to this toolkit to reinspire those strengths.

2) "Am I feeling slightly overwhelmed (or even completely untethered) as to how to harness the many ideas and desires swirling within my mind?"

If YES, practice **ROOT CHAKRA** flows and meditations to bring those inspirations and intentions back down to earth. (As mentioned above, the combo of Third Eye and Root Chakra is pretty much always recommended to capitalize on the idea process.)

3) "Am I finding myself spending too much time in arenas that are not fully encompassing the passion behind my vision?"

If YES, practice HEART CHAKRA flows and meditations to bring

yourself into an authentic place within your own heart where a know
ing will unfold and establish a framework for manifestation. (Affirm
that you are centered and focused in targeting your vision.)

*As always, no matter which energy field we are currently engaging, it is impor
tant to hold your intention in both mind and heart and then be open to the
inspiration that follows.*

ENERGY TYPES

ESTJ (Extraverted-Sensing-Thinking-Judger) - All Squared Away

If you are looking for someone to bring a sense of organization to your home, workplace, neighborhood, city or state, enter the ESTJ, pen, paper and agenda in hand. While most Judgers (Js) are into keeping track of life with a list, this type could possibly take the cake. They will make a list for themselves and everyone around them to insure that "We're all on the same wavelength." As a dominant Thinker (T), it's just the logical way to do things and also save some precious time. Being extraverted as well, the written word will not be their only form of task management. Usually quite adept at holding conferences, whether that be in the office or at the home kitchen table, they will keep all T's crossed and all I's dotted. (Their co-captain, Sensing - S - is quite adept at keeping these more minor details covered.)

Rules and regulations are part and parcel of the ESTJ's life and they are well aware that there is a standard way of achieving most anything one sets out to do. Just stick to the plan and you will be in control. Oh, but look out if someone, something or life in general throws a monkey wrench in the proposed line-up. All I can say, is if YOU are responsible for the change in plans, make your announcement as succinctly as possible... and run for it.

While this need for structure can be somewhat stifling to those more spontaneous folks in the lives of the ESTJ, it is also a reason that they are quite successful at any undertaking they set out to accomplish. Drive and ambition are just part of their makeup and they expect the same of their family members and employees.

The ESTJ is quite drawn to belonging to social clubs and associations and will often find themselves either at the helm or at least as part of the hierarchy of the group. Their innate sense of order is a sought-after commodity in most organizations.

This type also has a distinct love of tradition and will see to it that customs and beliefs are passed down from generation to generation.

When the ESTJ finds themselves undergoing a more than 'normal' amount of stress, they may initially become even more hard-nosed, which, should the stress escalate, could turn to somewhat of a melt down. Seeking solitude, options and alternatives (and not always the most logical) and experiencing a low level of depression could be the outcome if the world becomes too topsy-turvy.

In an intimate relationship, the ESTJ will usually take things step by step, allowing the natural flow of feelings to establish itself. When the time is right and a commitment is made, you can usually rest assured that this type will take it very seriously. Not always the most romantic of the types, they will, though, be there for you through hell and high water (rule book in hand.) The children of the ESTJ will know as much security and stability as is humanly possbile considering life circumstances, as this is the responsible way to raise a family.

Careerwise, the ESTJ will find their niche in an atmosphere where organization and structure are the key components. Military, management, educational institutions, and banking come to mind.

Responsible, reliable and traditional, the ESTJ adds the cornerstone to the structure of our world.

HIERARCHY OF FUNCTION ("Who's On First?")

The middle two letters of a person's type - our 'functions' - will equate to how we experience (perceive) reality and how we make our decisions. The 'authority' as to which of these processes occurs first will vary by type. There is an order we go through when accessing them and this is pretty much determined by the 'comfort zones' of our individual type.

We each have...
a DOMINANT FUNCTION (Team Captain)
an AUXILIARY FUNCTION (Co-captain)
a TERTIARY FUNCTION (Third at bat)
and an INFERIOR FUNCTION (Benchwarmer)

Of note, the Extravert (E) will 'share' their dominant process with the world and internalize their auxiliary. The Introvert (I) will do the opposite, keeping their most preferred function internal and showing the world the 'next in command.'

This is the breakdown fo the ESTJ:
DOMINANT (extraverted) T
AUXILIARY (introverted) S
TERTIARY (extraverted) N
INFERIOR (introverted) F

Type Preference by Letter for the ESTJ:

E/I (Extraversion /Introversion): *How we are energized...* If you choose **Extraversion** over Introversion, you are usually most energized when being in the company of others and sharing ideas. This does not mean that the E doesn't also require some quiet time. But having TOO much alone time for TOO long a period will be draining and the 'recharging process' will probably require some social interaction. Most Es will also talk their way through to making a point or coming to a decision as the entire thought process will be out in the open for all to hear. Now there exists a danger in this 'rambling' in that it could prove to be just that... rambling. Always confirm with an E exactly what you are hearing them say, especially if it involves YOU in any way just to make sure they aren't just venting aloud. The E may also have a hard time understanding why the I doesn't function in this same way and get frustrated when they need to play 'mind-reader.'

S/N (Sensing/iNtuition): *How we perceive reality...* This preference boils down to how we take in information, a vital component in communication. If we are experiencing *different* realities, learning to see things through the eyes of the receiving party will enable us to share in a way that will be understood. If you choose **Sensing** over iNtuition, you are probably very engaged in the world of detail, the past and day-to-day experience. Living in the present and in the tactile world of the five senses - i.e. what you see, hear, taste, smell and touch - is your reality and you are quite attuned to your environment. (This in comparison to the iNtuitive who resides in the realm of possibilities, trusts 'gut feelings' over past experience, is future-oriented and not always cognizant of what is going on in the physical world.

They tend to live beyond the 5 senses.) Being practical and dealing with 'what is' as opposed to 'what could be' are key attributes of the Sensing Type. The S may also take things quite literally which the N should keep in mind when sharing information as miscommunication *could* run rampant. ("You SAID be here on the hour... but you DIDN'T say which one!") All in all, they can make great partners, but understanding the different modes of perception is essential.

T/F (Thinking/Feeling): *How we make our decisions...* These are both rational means of decision-making but one will almost always offer a much more natural approach. When **Thinking** is preferred over Feeling (again please recall that these are Jungian terms and don't indicate that we don't all do both) the decisions will be more from the head than the heart i.e. the T tends to take an objective stance apart from the situation vs becoming embedded in the process. While we all practice both modes of determination and one will be more natural, it is highly beneficial to learn to look at both sides of an issue, subjectively as well as objectively. In the world of the Feeler, this is where things like "constructive criticism" become an oxymoron. If you are critical of an F from any standpoint, you can almost be certain they will be hurt. One of the biggest gifts the MBTI® offers, is the understanding of *why* we process certain things the way we do. For example, in this situation, the Feeler could learn that yes, it is okay to decide with your heart, but don't forget to balance it out by taking a step back and viewing the situation from the perspective of an observer. This is also helpful when dealing with Thinkers who may appear harsh or overly critical. Once it's understood that this is a decision making PROCESS, and not meant to be accusatory, these two preference types can come to a much better understanding. (The same being true for the Thinker dealing with the Feeler: "Why do you take everything to heart?") In truth, as in all preference pairings, we can learn so much from one another.

J/P (Judging/Perceiving): *Our lifestyle...* Choosing **Judging** over Perceiving usually indicates a preference for closure, structure and lists. "Let's wrap it up" could be the motto of most Js. Open ends tend to make them uncomfortable. Now many times, especially for the Feeling Judger, this could mean coming to closure just to avoid hurt feelings or any kind of conflict. (Which, depending on the situation, means you may end up having to deal with the scenario all over again.) This is in contrast to the P who prefers flexibility and leaving the door open until all options have been studied (or playing what I refer to as "ostrich." This entails putting your head in the ground and avoiding the fact that a decision even needs to be made.) Judgers like to live by a list and get a sense of achievement with crossing something off of that list. When living with a P, they may become critical if things aren't returned to their original place and also wonder why the P can't make simple decisions. (And the J knows exactly which way the TP and paper towels should come over the roll.) All in all, the J can lend structure and stability to just about any situation, and this is a wonderful trait, as long as they remain open to allowing for inevitable change.

ESTJ, CHAKRAS & BALANCE

I will now acquaint you with suggested toolkits for the **ESTJ** that will include specific yoga postures, breathing practices (Pranayama) meditations, affirmations, and mudras (seals or 'hand yoga).

After an explanation of the 'toolkits' I have chosen to help enhance and maintain your natural strength as well as regain balance when necessary, there will be a short series of questions you can ask yourself to clarify just which energy field is most in need of attention.

Suggested Toolkits to Celebrate, Nurture & Restore Balance:
Root Chakra, Third Eye Chakra, Heart Chakra

(Depending on your particular life situation, ANY of the chakras may 'deserve' attention. You can determine this by reviewing the questions found in each toolkit.)

As a dominant Thinker (T) combined with co-captain Sensing (S) AND Judging (J) preference, your strengths are found in your stability and groundedness. Working with the **ROOT CHAKRA TOOLKIT** will support those innate gifts and allow you to make the most of them. This is also a flow you can turn to if you are feeling LESS than grounded, in order to reestablish that footing.

While your natural inclinations will celebrate your ability to provide support and foundations within your life, you may also find spending time in the **THIRD EYE CHAKRA TOOLKIT** to be beneficial. Embrace this internal realm, especially if you are in the middle of any situation that demands relying on your intuition. 'Ajna' will make sure that you are seeing the whole picture and taking various possibilities into account. This will prevent coming to closure too soon which can quickly turn a decision into a 'whoops' moment.

Being a dominant Thinker (T) also gives rise to the benefit of spending time in the **HEART CHAKRA TOOLKIT.** This flow will provide you with the ability to see things from the perspective of who is being affected by your actions. Heart-based logic can equip you with a more centered, all-encompassing viewpoint when making your decisions.

All types need to be cognizant of the role that the throat chakra plays in our ability to communicate. The E-T will need to be wary of blurting out an opinion that may not actually be representative of what they are really feeling at all. But once it's out there, it's hard to take it back and the damage could already be done.

Questions for the ESTJ to ask themselves to determine which Chakra to nurture:

1) "Am I feeling grounded and able to support the current situations in my life??"

If YES, practice ROOT CHAKRA flows and meditations with the intention of connecting to earth energy and your ability to provide foundation. If NO, practice ROOT CHAKRA toolkit offerings to help bring you back into a your natural gifts of stability.

2) "Do I sense a need to explore beyond the daily list of to-dos and access a deeper sense of inner vision?"

If YES, practice THIRD EYE CHAKRA flows and meditations to embrace the innate sense of intuition that is available to us all when we bring our focus inward. Turn off the static of the outside world as you affirm the guidance that will come when you access this place of knowing.

3) "Am I feeling immersed in 'left-brain' analysis and needing to view things from a more subjetive viewpoint?"

If YES, practice HEART CHAKRA flows and meditations to open your heart space to the repercussions that your actions and decisions can cause.

As always, no matter which energy field we are currently engaging, it is important to hold your intention in both mind and heart and then be open to the inspirations that follow.

ENERGY TYPES

ESFJ (Extraverted-Sensing-Feeling-Judger) - My Home Is Your Home

You may be in the presence of an ESFJ if you hear, "Have you had enough to eat?" or "How is the temperature in here? Do I need to adjust the thermostat?" They will make sure your feet are warm and you have had your quota of hugs, encouragement or cookies for the day. In the workplace, they will keep the break room supplied in snacks and will be there the day after Thanksgiving to start the holiday decorating. Because they prefer to live their life according to a list and a calendar, you can also pretty much count on them to be punctual and precise.

Structure is a sought after commodity in the world of the ESFJ and they are most comfortable in a domain that's run with rules and boundaries. They may shy away from doing things in new and different ways as change is not always that welcome, especially if uninvited. Why stir up the pot if everything seems to be functioning just fine as is? But the danger zone here is that 'just fine' may be a figment of their wistful imagination. What it REALLY might be boiling down to is that it feels safer and less dramatic to stick with the status quo, even if it 'ain't perfect,' than to head off into unexplored realms and be totally out of the comfort zone.

Decision-making for the ESFJ will almost always revolve around WHO will be affected and how that will impact the lives of those involved. If life circumstances are in a demanding phase, they could easily go into the role of 'know-it-all' rescuer i.e. "I know what's best for you. Let me fix you." And THEN, if this advice/guidance is rebuffed, a wall could be erected that will require more than a gentle tipping over. (This can also lead to martyr-like reactions.) Add to this the ESFJ's mode of perception which is based on the 'here and now' and sensory input, and chances are, whatever is shared will undoubtedly be taken literally.

When you enter the home of an ESFJ, it will most likely reflect the order that they so cherish in their lifestyle: Clean, tidy and almost certainly color-coordinated (as their clothing tends to be as well... even down to the undies.) This orderliness brings with it a sense of deep satisfaction as well as security AND they will almost always be able to find anything they are looking for, because THEY put things back where they belong. (Hear that Ps?)

In the arena of business and career, ESFJs tend toward service-oriented positions such as teaching (usually younger grades for more 'hands-on"instruction vs. theory), ministerial work, or medical fields such as nursing or physician assistants. In any case, the environment should support the E's need for interaction, as being in a solitary mode for too long a time could result in stress associated with not being able to share thoughts and ideas.

In intimate relationships, the ESFJ looks for a partnership that reflects the core essense of dedication. They can often put the needs of a partner (as well as children) before themselves, which if taken to an extreme, can lead to resentment. Loyalty is a huge part of their 'repertoire' and they tend to expect this level of commitment in return.

The ESFJ under stress will first become even more rigid. Then, if pushed even further, may adopt a completely uncharacteristic devil-may-care attitude, while at the same time furiously researching options and alternatives to get them out of this mess. This, though, rather than solving the dilemma usually just causes even further confusion and on it goes... As groundedness and security are the hallmarks of this type, spinning out of control is an area that is quite foreign to them.

Overall, this type feels most complete and fulfilled when those close to them are fulfilled as well. Ever ready to be of service, the ESFJ offers the world a caring shoulder.

HIERARCHY OF FUNCTION ("Who's On First?")

The middle two letters of a person's type - our 'functions' - will equate to how we experience (perceive) reality and how we make our decisions. The 'authority' as to which of these processes occurs first will vary by type. There is an order we go through when accessing them and this is pretty much determined by the 'comfort zones' of our individual type.

We each have...
a DOMINANT FUNCTION (Team Captain)
an AUXILIARY FUNCTION (Co-captain)
a TERTIARY FUNCTION (Third at bat)
and an INFERIOR FUNCTION (Benchwarmer)

Of note, the Extravert (E) will 'share' their dominant process with the world and internalize their auxiliary. The Introvert (I) will do the opposite, keeping their most preferred function internal and showing the world the 'next in command.'

This is the breakdown fo the ESFJ:
DOMINANT (extraverted) F
AUXILIARY (introverted)) S
TERTIARY (extraverted) N
INFERIOR (introverted) T

Type Preference by Letter for the ESFJ:

E/I (Extraversion /Introversion): *How we are energized...* If you choose **Extraversion** over Introversion, you are usually most energized when being in the company of others and sharing ideas. This does not mean that the E doesn't also require some quiet time. But having TOO much alone time for TOO long a period will be draining and the 'recharging process' will probably require some social interaction. Most Es will also talk their way through to making a point or coming to a decision as the entire thought process will be out in the open for all to hear. Now there exists a danger in this 'rambling' in that it could prove to be just that... rambling. Always confirm with an E exactly what you are hearing them say, especially if it involves YOU in any way just to make sure they aren't just venting aloud. The E may also have a hard time understanding why the I doesn't function in this same way and get frustrated when they need to play 'mind-reader.'

S/N (Sensing/iNtuition): *How we perceive reality...* This preference boils down to how we perceive reality, which is indeed a vital component in communication. If we are experiencing *different* realities,learning to see things through the eyes of the receiving party will enable us to share in a way that will be understood. If you choose **Sensing** over iNtuition, you are probably very engaged in the world of detail, the past and day-to-day experience. Living in the present and in the tactile world of the five senses - i.e. what you see, hear, taste, smell and touch - is your reality and you are quite attuned to your environment. (This in comparison to the iNtuitive who resides in the realm of possibilities, trusts 'gut feelings' over past experience, is future-oriented and not always cognizant of what is going on in the physical world. They tend to live beyond the 5 senses.) Being practical and dealing with 'what is' as opposed to 'what could be' are key attributes of the Sensing Type. The S may also take things quite literally which the N should keep in mind when sharing information as miscommunication *could* run rampant. ("You SAID be here on the hour... but you DIDN'T say which one!") All in all, they can make great partners, but understanding the different modes of perception is essential.

T/F (Thinking/Feeling): *How we make our decisions...* If you choose **Feeling** over Thinking as your method of decision making, you tend to become embedded in the situation you are currently encountering. While we all practice both modes of determination, this arena will most often be a more comfortable fit for you. And though one will feel more natural, it is highly beneficial to learn to look at both sides of an issue, subjectively as well as objectively. In the world of the Feeler, this is where things like "constructive criticism" become an oxymoron. If you are critical of an F from any standpoint, you can almost be certain they will be hurt. One of the biggest gifts the MBTI® offers, is the understanding of *why* we process certain things the way we do. For example, in this situation, the Feeler could learn that yes, it is okay to decide with your heart, but don't forget to balance it out by taking a step backward and viewing thesituation from the per-spective of an observer. This is also helpful when dealing with Thinkers who may appear harsh or overly critical. Once it's under stood that this is a decision making PROCESS, and not meant to be accusatory, these two preference types can come to much better understanding. (The same being true for the Thinker dealing with the Feeler: "Why do you take everything to heart?") In truth, as in all preference pairings, we can learn so much from one another.

J/P (Judging/Perceiving): *Our lifestyle...* Choosing **Judging** over Perceiving usually indicates a preference for closure, structure and lists. "Let's wrap it up" could be the motto of most Js. Open ends tend to make them uncomfortable. Now many times, especially for the Feeling Judger, this could mean coming to closure just to avoid hurt feelings or any kind of conflict. (Which means, depending on the situation, you may end up having to deal with the scenario all over again.) This is in contrast to the P who prefers flexibility and leaving the door open until all options have been studied (or playing what I refer to as "ostrich." This entails putting your head in the ground and avoiding the fact that a decision even needs to be made.) Judgers like to live by a list and get a sense of achievement with crossing something off of that list. When living with a P, they may become critical if things aren't returned to their original place and also wonder why the P can't make simple decisions. (And the J knows exactly which way the TP and paper towels should come over the roll.) All in all, the J can lend structure and stability to just about any situation, and this is a wonderful trait, as long as they remain open to allowing for inevitable change.

ESFJ, CHAKRAS & BALANCE

I will now acquaint you with suggested toolkits for the **ESFJ** that will include specific yoga postures, breathing practices (Pranayama) meditations, affirmations, and mudras (seals or 'hand yoga).

After an explanation of the 'toolkits' I have chosen to help enhance and maintain your natural strength as well as regain balance when necessary, there will be a short series of questions you can ask your-self to clarify just which energy field is most in need of attention.

Suggested Toolkits to Celebrate, Nurture & Restore Balance:
Heart Chakra, Solar Plexus Chakra, Sacral Chakra

(Depending on your particular life situation, ANY of the chakras may 'deserve' attention. You can determine this by reviewing the questions found in each toolkit.)

As a dominant Feeler ("team captain" of your type) the heart chakra will be your home playing field. When life is flowing along in a healthy state, the **HEART CHAKRA TOOLKIT** is where you can go to not only help maintain that balance, but to celebrate your gifts of empathy, compassion and heart-based leadership.

This is also the flow you may choose to practice if you ask yourself the question, "Am I feeling depleted?" and the answer is 'yes.' This would be in cases of perhaps going through a period of grief or hav-ing given so much of yourself due to life circumstances that you find yourself needing a dose of heart chakra nourishment. This will allow you to open up both sides of the heart - able to give, but also able to receive and keep the energy circulating.

On the other hand if you are depleted due to an enabling situation, especially if you find yourself experiencing feelings of resentment, you will need to turn to your inferior function ("last to be asked to join the party") and in the case of the ESFJ, that refers to the Thinking Function and the **SOLAR PLEXUS TOOLKIT**. When the heart energy field is weakened or drained, we need to build up feelings of courage, confidence and self-esteem so that the playing field is leveled once again.

Under healthy conditions, the S-J (Sensing-Judging) part of your personality is quite capable of keeping you feeling grounded and stable. If you do become fearful, this could become magnified and rather than offer security, have you holding on so tight that you feel like you are standing in quicksand. The antidote? Movement! Enter the **SACRAL CHAKRA TOOLKIT**.... all about the water element of flow, desire, relationship to self and others and getting the ball rolling. Turn here whenever you are feeling 'stuck in the muck' and bogged down by life.

All types need to be cognizant of the role that the throat chakra plays in our ability to communicate. The E-F will need to be wary of either suppressing truth in the interest of not hurting anyone's feelings or sugar coating a situation that is in need of honest communcation. This is at the expense of their own health and personal truth.

Questions for the ESFJ to ask themselves to determine which Chakra to nurture:

1) "Am I in a position where my heart is leading the way and I feel strong and giving?"

If YES, practice HEART CHAKRA TOOLKIT flows to maintain this sense of heart-felt leadership. If NO, due to depletion through grief or inability to receive the love you deserve, turn to this toolkit as well.

2) *"Are feelings of low self worth or loss of confidence keeping me from moving forward and achieving my goals?"* OR *"Are my rescuing tendencies leaving me resentful and running on empty?"*

If YES, practice SOLAR PLEXUS CHAKRA flows and meditations to increase the confidence and vigor within yourself. This 'fire' will reignite feelings of personal power that are necessary not only to enable you to practice self-care, but to continue to share love with others in your life from a healthy, balanced place.

3) *"Do I feel the weight of the world on my shoulders and unable to 'get in the flow'?"*

If YES, practice SACRAL CHAKRA flows and meditations to introduce the water element into your life. Allow desire, movement, and the planting of seeds in the fertile soil of the root chakra to reinvigorate you and spur you on to new beginnings.

As always, no matter which energy field we are currently engaging, it is important to hold your intention in both mind and heart and then be open to the inspiration that follows.

ENERGY TYPES

ENFJ (Extraverted-Intuitive-Feeling-Judger) - Here to Liberate the World

*A*nyone out there need rescuing? Or at least a guide book containing some pertinent information on how you can then ALSO help save the world? Enter the ENFJ. Determining a life purpose is of supreme importance to most ENFJs as they make their way along their earthly path. They will most likely assume that this should be a goal of yours as well and are consistently bewildered by those who aren't seeking that calling.

Communicating what they 'know to be true' comes easily as their comfort in talking to others (ordinarily with a somewhat persuasive bent) is a natural characteristic of their extraverted personality. Whether they meet you in line at the grocery store or in a parking garage elevator, they will attempt to at least make eye contact. If they sense approval, they will then share a comment about anything happening to be going through their iNuitive mind at the time. (This usually in the hopes of making you smile.)

At the helm for this type is dominant Feeling and their first stop in almost any situation will be this subjective decision-making mode. Their extraversion accounts for this readily apparent wearing of the heart on their sleeve. I would be willing to bet that many of the non-profit organizations in existence today that support the underprivileged (whether that be human or beast) have at least one ENFJ at the wheel. And beware the soapbox: If the ENFJ feels that someone (of

181

any life form) is being wronged, they will make it their job to personally inform anyone within an accessible radius, which, of course,
with the scope of the internet, means the world. (They also carry a
megaphone with them at all times. Just in case.)

As is indeed the case with most dominant Feelers, they can find
themselves in the role of 'giver' and not often enough in the role of
'receiver.' (This can, of course, be their own doing.) But what often
results from this behavior, is that not only do others come to expect
this royal treatment, they themselves begin to feel resentful of other's
expectations. If they would take a step back, they would realize it was
their own penchant for keeping everyone happy that brought about
this scenario in the first place.

Being a Judger (J) keeps them somewhat organized and structured.
Calendars are their friend as their social life, between work and play,
is normally quite full. (They also prefer to look at WORK as play
even if it isn't always that much fun. Better attitude, you know?)
This sense of organization may sometimes not be readily visible
because as an iNtuitive, they also live in a world of possibilities.
Making leaps from one subject to the next will be a natural activity
for them and if you aren't quite 'tuned in' to their frequency, they can
appear a bit scattered. But hey, with the number of people and animals that need saving out there, they had better be ready to switch
gears when necessary.

Career-wise, then, it is not surprising that they often choose service-
oriented professions such as teaching, motivational speaking or healing type avenues of expression. This is especially true in today's
world where energy medicine is becoming more and more accepted
and sought after.

182

In intimate relationships, the ENFJ is a true romantic and will throw their entire heart into the ring. But while more than willing to be devoted and caring partners, they also still desire their independence. If they begin to feel 'fenced in,' this could bring about an air of aloofness as they attempt to reestablish their own individuality.

Charismatic, sometimes stubborn but willing to do whatever it takes to 'free the repressed'... that's the ENFJ.

HIERARCHY OF FUNCTION ("Who's On First?")

The middle two letters of a person's type - our 'functions' - will equate to how we experience (perceive) reality and how we make our decisions. The 'authority' as to which of these processes occurs first will vary by type. There is an order we go through when accessing them and this is pretty much determined by the 'comfort zones' of our individual type.

We each have...

a DOMINANT FUNCTION (Team Captain)
an AUXILIARY FUNCTION (Co-captain)
a TERTIARY FUNCTION (Third at bat)
and an INFERIOR FUNCTION (Benchwarmer)

Of note, the Extravert (E) will 'share' their dominant process with the world and internalize their auxiliary. The Introvert (I) will do the opposite, keeping their most preferred function internal and showing the world the 'next in command.'

This is the breakdown for the ENFJ:

DOMINANT (extraverted) F
AUXILIARY (introverted) N
TERTIARY (extraverted) S
INFERIOR (introverted) T

Type Preference by Letter for the ENFJ:

E/I (Extraversion /Introversion): *How we are energized...* If you choose **Extraversion** over Introversion, you are usually most energized when being in the company of others and sharing ideas. This does not mean that the E doesn't also require some quiet time. But having TOO much alone time for TOO long a period will be draining and the 'recharging process' will probably require some social interaction. Most Es will also talk their way through to making a point or coming to a decision as the entire thought process will be out in the open for all to hear. Now there exists a danger in this 'rambling' in that it could prove to be just that... rambling. Always confirm with an E exactly what you are hearing them say, especially if it involves YOU in any way just to make sure they aren't just venting aloud. The E may also have a hard time understanding why the I doesn't function in this same way and get frustrated when they need to play 'mind-reader.'

S/N (Sensing/iNtuition): *How we gather information...* This preference boils down to how we perceive reality, which is indeed a vital component in communication. If we are experiencing *different* realities, learning to see things through the eyes of the receiving party will enable us to share in a way that will be understood. Choosing **iNtuition** over Sensing indicates being engaged in the world of possibilities, trusting gut feelings over past experience, looking to the future vs. what is currently 'on the table', and therefore not always being totally cognizant of what is going on right in front of one's nose. (e.g. walking right by something without seeing it if they aren't looking for it. And actually, sometimes even then). This is in contrast to the Sensor's comfort zone in the 'here and now' and trusting of five senses over conjecture.

T/F (Thinking/Feeling): *How we make our decisions...* If you choose **Feeling** over Thinking as your method of decision making, you tend to become embedded in the situation you are currently encountering. While we all practice both modes of determination, this arena will most often be a more comfortable fit for you. And though one will feel more natural, it is highly beneficial to learn to look at both sides of an issue, subjectively as well as objectively. In the world of the Feeler, this is where things like "constructive criticism" become an oxymoron. If you are critical of an F from any standpoint, you can almost be certain they will be hurt. One of the biggest gifts the MBTI® offers, is the understanding of *why* we process certain things the way we do. For example, in this situation, the Feeler could learn that yes, it is okay to decide with your heart, but don't forget to balance it out by taking a step back and viewing the situation from the perspective of an observer. This is also helpful when dealing with Thinkers who may appear harsh or overly critical. Once it's understood that this is a decision making PROCESS, and not meant to be accusatory, these two preference types can come to much better understanding. (The same being true for the Thinker dealing with the Feeler: "Why do you take everything to heart?") In truth, as in all preference pairings, we can learn so much from one another.

J/P (Judging/Perceiving): *Our lifestyle...* Choosing **Judging** over Perceiving usually indicates a preference for closure, structure and lists. "Let's wrap it up" could be the motto of most Js. Open ends tend to make them uncomfortable. Now many times, especially for the Feeling Judger, this could mean coming to closure just to avoid hurt feelings or any kind of conflict. (Which, depending on the situation, means you may end up having to deal with the scenario all over again.) This is in contrast to the P who prefers flexibility and leaving the door open until all options have been studied (or playing what I refer to as "ostrich." This entails putting your head in the ground and avoiding the fact that a decision even needs to be made.) Judgers like to live by a list and get a sense of achievement with crossing something off of that list. When living with a P, they may become critical if things aren't returned to their original place and also wonder why the P can't make simple decisions. (And the J knows exactly which way the TP and paper towels should come over the roll.) All in all, the J can lend structure and stability to just about any situation, and this is a wonderful trait, as long as they remain open to allowing for inevitable change.

ENFJ, CHAKRAS & BALANCE

I will now acquaint you with suggested toolkits for the **ENFJ** that will include specific yoga postures, breathing practices (Pranayama) meditations, affirmations, and mudras (seals or 'hand yoga).

After an explanation of the 'toolkits' I have chosen to help enhance and maintain your natural strength as well as regain balance when necessary, there will be a short series of questions you can ask yourself to clarify just which energy field is most in need of attention.

Suggested Toolkits to Celebrate,
Nurture & Restore Balance:
Heart Chakra, Solar Plexus Chakra,
Root Chakra

(Depending on your particular life situation, ANY of the chakras may 'deserve' attention. You can determine this by reviewing the questions found in each toolkit.)

As a dominant Feeler ("team captain" of your type) the heart chakra will be your home playing field. When life is flowing along in a healthy state, the **HEART CHAKRA TOOLKIT** is where you can go to not only help maintain that balance, but to celebrate your gifts of empathy, compassion and heart-based leadership. Humanitarian causes, here you come! This is also the flow you may choose to practice if you ask yourself the question, "Am I feeling depleted?" and the answer is 'yes.' This would be in cases of perhaps going through a period of grief or having given so much of yourself due to life circumstances that you find yourself needing a dose of heart chakra nourishment. This will allow you to open up both sides of the heart - able to give, but also able to receive and keep the energy circulating.

On the other hand if you are depleted due to an enabling situation, especially if you find yourself experiencing feelings of resentment, you will need to turn to your Inferior function ("last to be asked to join the party") and in the case of the ENFJ, that refers to the Thinking function and the **SOLAR PLEXUS TOOLKIT**. When the heart energy field is weakened or drained, we need to build up feelings of courage, confidence and self-esteem so that the playing field is leveled once again.

When the ENFJ is on a roll (easy to recognize... their soap box can be seen from a mile away) they can be so filled with bringing their cause to fruition that their feet don't touch the ground anymore. In the interest of being reeled back into the world of matter, spending time in **ROOT CHAKRA TOOLKIT** can assure that the manifestation of your brainstorm has a much better chance of taking place. Also, try including a morning run or walk each day or just being out in nature and feeling your footfall on the earth to tremendously augment this grounding influence.

All types need to be cognizant of the role that the throat chakra plays in our ability to communicate. The E-F will need to be wary of suppressing truth in the interest of not hurting anyone's feelings or of sharing what they think the other person wants to hear just to smooth everything out (but not really); this at the expense of their own health and personal integrity.

Questions for the ENFJ to ask themselves to determine which Chakra to nurture:

1) *"Am I in a position where my heart is leading the way and I feel strong and giving?"*

If YES, practice HEART CHAKRA flows to maintain this sense of heart-felt leadership. If NO, due to depletion through grief or inability to receive the love you deserve, turn to this toolkit as well.

2) *"Have I reached a point where I am sponge for other people's pain and feel unable to voice my frustration?"*

If YES, practice SOLAR PLEXUS CHAKRA flows and meditations to increase the confidence and vigor within yourself. This 'fire' will reignite feelings of personal power that are necessary not only to enable you to practice self-care, but to continue to share love with others in your life from a healthy, balanced place.

3) Are you so immersed in the possibilities and aspirations behind your 'mankind enhancing' project that turning it into reality is feeling elusive?

If YES, turn to the ROOT CHAKRA TOOLKIT to reestabish your connection to the grounding of the earth element.

As always, no matter which energy field we are currently engaging, it is important to hold your intention in both mind and heart and then be open to the inspiration that follows.

ENERGY TYPES

ENTJ (Extraverted Intuitive Thinking Judger) - Onward and Upward

The ENTJ probably learned in nursery school or perhaps as late as kindergarten that they had an innate gift to lead and not in a traditional sense mind you, but in a way that would introduce the other children to thinking outside the sandbox. Those that didn't follow along probably watched in awe as the other children learned to do things in new and different ways (possibly causing the occasional raised eyebrow among the teachers.)

As a dominant Thinker, the ENTJ begins most of their decision-making journeys from the land of objectivity and then travels to the universe of possibilities. They are apt to be sharing their ideas along the way and will most likely bring them to closure quite rapidly (whether you agree with their conclusions or not.)

Innovative and resourceful, they make excellent team managers and are more than willing to integrate entirely new methodologies if need be. Sticking to the tried and true is not a big deal to the ENTJ and to be honest, probably quite a boring prospect. They would prefer to discover new and unique ways to tackle any situation.

With that in mind, they could definitely have a tendency to want to improve on the status quo in any scenario and will not hesitate to let you know that. These improvements may or may not be necessary in the eyes of the person being impacted or in consideration of the situation being improved upon.

An evident characteristic of most ENTJs is their independent nature. Despite this, or even because of it, they will usually also desire feedback on their various endeavors. If these reviews are deemed unfavorable, they may not take too kindly to what will possibly be perceived as criticism, though they will still bear it in mind. If they are convinced there is, in fact, room for improvement, they will be the first to escalate their efforts.

The ENTJ under stress can adopt a rather negative outlook. Their perfectionist leanings are aimed not only at the outside world but rather strictly at themselves as well. If they don't live up to their own standards of excellence, you may witness quite the harsh self-criticism.

As competition in any packaging can be quite attractive to the ENTJ, the same could hold true in intimate relationships. The idea of 'pursuit' i.e. attracting a partner who is playing hard to get, will just make the game that much more enjoyable. Having something handed over on a silver platter could diminish the value in their estimation. (If you have indeed fallen for an ENTJ, my suggestion would be make them work for it and enjoy the quest.) Tradition is probably not real high on the scale of importance for this type, though it does have its place. They would prefer to take an age-old tradition and 'tweak' it just to see what might happen. (For instance, "What if we celebrated Thanksgiving in February in conjunction with Valentine's Day? Love and gratitude all on one day!")

Typical career choices may include sales, law, architecture (avant-garde), upper management and areas that are on the cutting edge (energy work for example.)

Unique, hard-working, dedicated and forward-thinking, the ENTJ is a leader in every sense of the word.

HIERARCHY OF FUNCTION ("Who's On First?")

The middle two letters of a person's type - our 'functions' - will equate to how we experience (perceive) reality and how we make our decisions. The 'authority' as to which of these processes occurs first will vary by type. There is an order we go through when accessing them and this is pretty much determined by the 'comfort zones' of our individual type.

We each have...
a DOMINANT FUNCTION (Team Captain)
an AUXILIARY FUNCTION (Co-captain)
a TERTIARY FUNCTION (Third at bat)
and an INFERIOR FUNCTION (Benchwarmer)

Of note, the Extravert (E) will 'share' their dominant process with the world and internalize their auxiliary. The Introvert (I) will do the opposite, keeping their most preferred function internal and showing the world the 'next in command.'

This is the breakdown fo the ENTJ:
DOMINANT (extraverted) T
AUXILIARY (introverted) N
TERTIARY (extraverted) S
INFERIOR (introverted) F

Type Preference by Letter for the ENTJ:

E/I (**Extraversion** /Introversion): *How we are energized...* If you choose **Extraversion** over Introversion, you are usually most energized when being in the company of others and sharing ideas. This does not mean that the E doesn't also require some quiet time. But having TOO much alone time for TOO long a period will be draining and the 'recharging process' will probably require some social interaction. Most Es will also talk their way through to making a point or coming to a decision as the entire thought process will be out in the open for all to hear. Now there exists a danger in this 'rambling' in that it could prove to be just that... rambling. Always confirm with an E exactly what you are hearing them say, especially if it involves YOU in any way just to make sure they aren't just venting aloud. The E may also have a hard time understanding why the I doesn't function in this same way and get frustrated when they need to play 'mind-reader.'

S/N (**Sensing**/iNtuition): *How we gather information...* This preference boils down to how we take in information, a vital component in communication. If we are experiencing *different* realities, learning to see things through the eyes of the receiving party will enable us to share in a way that will be understood. Choosing **iNtuition** over Sensing indicates being engaged in the world of possibilities, trusting gut feelings over past experience, looking to the future vs. what is currently 'on the table', and therefore not always being totally cognizant of what is going on right in front of one's nose. (e.g. walking right by something without seeing it if they aren't looking for it. And actually, sometimes even then). This is in contrast to the Sensor's comfort zone in the 'here and now' and trusting of five senses over conjecture.

T/F (Thinking/Feeling): *How we make our decisions...* These are both rational means of decision-making but one will almost always offer a much more natural approach. When **Thinking** is preferred over Feeling (again please recall that these are Jungian terms and don't indicate that we don't all do both) the decisions will be more from the head than the heart i.e. the T tends to take an objective stance apart from the situation vs becoming embedded in the process. While we all practice both modes of determination and one will be more natural, it is highly beneficial to learn to look at both sides of an issue, subjectively as well as objectively. In the world of the Feeler, this is where things like "constructive criticism" become an oxymoron. If you are critical of an F from any standpoint, you can almost be certain they will be hurt. One of the biggest gifts the MBTI® offers, is the understanding of *why* we process certain things the way we do. For example, in this situation, the Feeler could learn that yes, it is okay to decide with your heart, but don't forget to balance it out by taking a step back and viewing the situation from the perspective of an observer. This is also helpful when dealing with Thinkers who may appear harsh or overly critical. Once it's understood that this is a decision making PROCESS, and not meant to be accusatory, these two preference types can come to much better understanding. (The same being true for the Thinker dealing with the Feeler: "Why do you take everything to heart?") In truth, as in all preference pairings, we can learn so much from one another.

J/P (Judging/Perceiving): *Our lifestyle...* Choosing **Judging** over Perceiving usually indicates a preference for closure, structure and lists. "Let's wrap it up" could be the motto of most Js. Open ends tend to make them uncomfortable. Now many times, especially for the Feeling Judger, this could mean coming to closure just to avoid hurt feelings or any kind of conflict. (Which means, depending on the situation, means you may end up having to deal with the scenario all over again.) This is in contrast to the P who prefers flexibility and leaving the door open until all options have been studied (or playing what I refer to as "ostrich." This entails putting your head in the ground and avoiding the fact that a decision even needs to be made.) Judgers like to live by a list and get a sense of achievement with crossing something off of that list. When living with a P, they may become critical if things aren't returned to their original place and also wonder why the P can't make simple decisions. (And the J knows exactly which way the TP and paper towels should come over the roll.) All in all, the J can lend structure and stability to just about any situation, and this is a wonderful trait, as long as they remain open to allowing for inevitable change.

ENTJ, CHAKRAS & BALANCE

I will now acquaint you with suggested toolkits for the **ENTJ** that will include specific yoga postures, breathing practices (Pranayama) meditations, affirmations, and mudras (seals or 'hand yoga).

After an explanation of the 'toolkits' I have chosen to help enhance and maintain your natural strength as well as regain balance when necessary, there will be a short series of questions you can ask yourself to clarify just which energy field is most in need of attention.

Suggested Toolkits to Celebrate, Nurture & Restore Balance:
Solar Plexus Chakra, Root Chakra, Heart Chakra

(Depending on your particular life situation, ANY of the chakras may 'deserve' attention. You can determine this by reviewing the questions found in each toolkit.)

The 'team captain' for the ENTJ, the Thinking function will be a realm of innate strength for you. In order to celebrate your natural leadership abilities, I would recommend practicing the flow and meditation found in the **SOLAR PLEXUS CHAKRA TOOLKIT**. If you find yourself especially passionate regarding a life goal, this will up the anty and stoke the fire within. (In this same vein, if the fire has become a little 'too hot to handle,' whether that be in relationship to home or to work, you may also consider turning to the **SACRAL CHAKRA TOOLKIT** and allow the water element to cool things down and resume a natural, even flow.)

Your 'co-captain', the iNtuitive function, will also prove key in supporting the visions behind your goals. This area can also cause us to get side-tracked in the realm of possibilities. Should this be the case, turning to the **ROOT CHAKRA TOOLKIT** will bring grounding to your endeavors by streamlining your intent.

When under more than normal stressful conditions, you may find yourself turning inward in what could be viewed as a melancholic manner. Practicing the flow and meditation found within the **HEART CHAKRA TOOLKIT** should assist you in bringing clarity to what is truly most important in your life and achieving your state of natural exhuberance.

All types need to be cognizant of the role that the throat chakra plays in our ability to communicate. The E-T will need to be wary of blurting out an opinion that may not actually be representative of what they are really feeling at all. But once it's out there, it's hard to take it back and the damage could already be done.

Questions for the ENTJ to ask themselves to determine which Chakra to nurture:

1) "Am I feeling passionate and enthusiastic about the goals in my life?"

If YES, practice SOLAR PLEXUS CHAKRA flows and meditations with the intention of honoring your innate gifts of leadership and trailblazing. If NO, then also turn to this toolkit to reinspire those strengths.

2) "Am I longing to put my project into action but experiencing a sense of confusion because I feel drawn in multiple directions?"

If YES, practice the ROOT CHAKRA flows and meditations to reestablish your sense of grounding.

3) "Have I been spending so much time in the manifesting of projects that the people in my life have been getting the short end of the stick?

If YES, practice HEART CHAKRA flows and meditations to bring yourself into an authentic place within your own heart regarding the truly important things in life.

As always, no matter which energy field we are currently engaging, it is important to hold your intention in both mind and heart and then be open to the inspiration that follows.

So now I dance,
sometimes fast, sometimes slow.
The sound of my heartbeat says
which way to go...
- Maureen

CHAPTER 4

Chakra Toolkits:
Yoga Poses, Breathing Practices, Meditations, Affirmations & Mudras

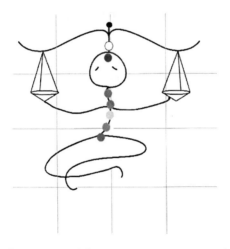

The description of the various yoga poses and flows offered in 'Energy Types' are general in nature. If you have any questions or concerns regarding the integrity, contraindications or preciseness of a pose, there are many wonderful references available online such as yogajournal.com.

Basic Needs At A Glance...

Sometimes by just identifying a basic need we can pinpoint where the scales are being tipped in a particular chakra. Answering the following questions can give you some quick guidance as to which toolkit would benefit you in your current situation.

1) Do I need grounding?
- Root Chakra

2) Do I need movement to inspire the creative process?
- Sacral Chakra

3) Do I need to increase my personal power?
- Solar Plexus Chakra

4) Do I need more compassion (for myself and/or others?)
- Heart Chakra

5) Do I need to speak my truth (with myself or others)?
- Throat Chakra

6) Do I need intuitive guidance?
- Third Eye Chakra

7) Do I need more trust in my connection to the Divine?
- Crown Chakra

Root Chakra Toolkit

Location: Base of Spine
Related Color: Red

When BALANCED... We feel a blessed connection with the earth beneath our feet, stable and deserving of our right to have and to be.

When we are grounded, we are able to find comfort in the present moment, knowing when to hold steady and also sensingwhen movement (change) is necessary.

When the SCALES ARE TIPPED...

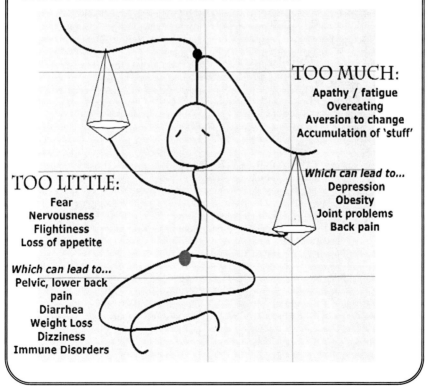

TOO MUCH:
Apathy / fatigue
Overeating
Aversion to change
Accumulation of 'stuff'

Which can lead to...
Depression
Obesity
Joint problems
Back pain

TOO LITTLE:
Fear
Nervousness
Flightiness
Loss of appetite

Which can lead to...
Pelvic, lower back pain
Diarrhea
Weight Loss
Dizziness
Immune Disorders

mindful walking
step by step
sensing ground underfoot
breath matching cadence...

wind dances in trees and
plays in my hair

sunshine warms my face
and melts my heart

moment by moment
a song emerges
a gentle symphony of the senses

how blessed i feel

choosing to be a grateful conduit
for nature's expression

this idyllic day.

- Maureen

ROOT CHAKRA -
MULADHARA ("ROOT SUPPORT")

*T*he first energy field, our root chakra, is located at the base of the spine and forms the foundation of our chakra system. Associated with the element of earth, our root chakra represents feelings of stability and belonging. If our footing is not stable, it is easy to understand how that can affect the rest of our life. This chakra is representative of our most basic survival instincts and can also reveal a predisposition regarding the belief system we are born into and passed down by generations preceding us. Family ties and primal needs are focal points of this energy field. "Muladhara" is also connected to the color red.

When our root chakra is in balance, we feel grounded, secure and in tune with Mother Earth. Like the roots of a tree, we feel connected and strong. If there is a weakness in this field, however, we may feel that the 'ground is literally moving under our feet' and the path before us will not be clear.

Here are some questions to ask yourself to determine your balance in the ROOT CHAKRA.

You may be Root Chakra deficient if you answer 'yes' to the following...

* *Am I feeling fearful or unstable regarding my life situation?*
* *Is my head spinning with possibilities that seem to lead nowhere?*
* *Is anxiety affecting my decision-making ability and eating habits?*
* *Have I lost touch with the beauty and splendor of Mother Nature?*

If you answered in the affirmative to any or all of the preceding questions, you are in exactly the right place because earth energy is calling. Working with the root chakra will help you reestablish your footing, celebrate your connection with Mother Earth and affirm your sense of security.

**You may be in Root Chakra excess if you answer
'yes' to the following:**

* Am I feeling so 'stuck in the muck' that there seem to be no options?
* Do I feel foggy and unable to tap into my intuition?
* Am I apathetic about my future and fearful of change?
* Am I either overeating or holding on to more stuff than I actually need?

If you responded in the positive to any of *these* questions, chances are you need to bring in some energy from other fields. The SACRAL CHAKRA TOOLKIT and the element of water will introduce flow and motion into your life and invite you to 'move your feet.' The THIRD EYE CHAKRA TOOLKIT can shift the energy up to the realm of intuition where your own inner wisdom will 'lighten' things up and open the door to new possibilities.

Root Chakra: Breathwork & Mudras

EARTH BREATH: Inhale and exhale through the nose, drawing energy up from Mother Earth, allowing her beautiful vitality to fill and ground you. As you exhale, allow tension and any feelings of lack or instability to be released from your body, but also in a gesture of giving back *through* your breath to our earth, mindful of our connection to one another. You can also picture *your* inhale being the EXHALE of the earth, taking in the energy of the wind, the ocean, the trees... and your exhale then becomes the INHALE of Mother Earth, as you fill her with your own love. A beautiful, mutually nurturing pattern of breath.

PRITHIVI MUDRA (EARTH MUDRA): Bring thumb and ring fingers together and allow other fingers to extend out in relaxed manner. This pose energizes the earth connection.

PRANA MUDRA (LIFE FORCE): Bring tips of thumb, ring finger and little finger together, others extended. This 'hand yoga' position is rejuvenating and will energize, increase vitality and decrease fatigue.

Root Chakra Intention:
Working with the following flow will help you to re-establish feelings of groundedness and connection. In addition to these poses, going out into nature, spending time in a forest, at the ocean or anywhere you can feel our beautiful earth beneath your feet, will reacquaint you with 'our right to have and to be.'

Affirmation for Root Chakra:
I am guided, protected and all of my needs are met.

ROOT CHAKRA FLOW

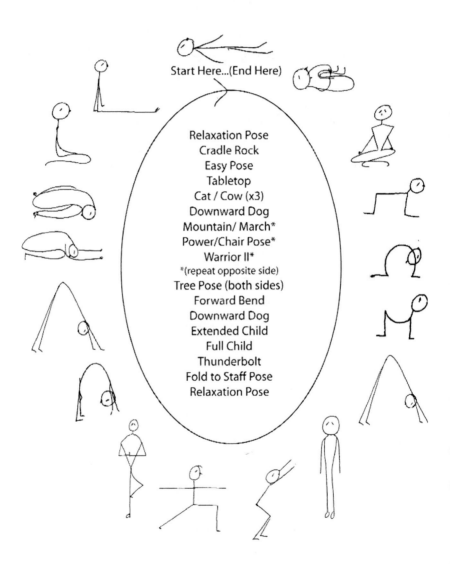

Start Here...(End Here)

Relaxation Pose
Cradle Rock
Easy Pose
Tabletop
Cat / Cow (x3)
Downward Dog
Mountain/ March*
Power/Chair Pose*
Warrior II*
*(repeat opposite side)
Tree Pose (both sides)
Forward Bend
Downward Dog
Extended Child
Full Child
Thunderbolt
Fold to Staff Pose
Relaxation Pose

Description of YOGA POSES for **Root Chakra Flow:**

As with all poses listed here in Energy Types, please modify to suit your own particular strength, flexibility and/or health challenges.

RELAXATION/CORPSE POSE (Savasana): Lying on back, eyes closed, arms and legs spead at about 45 degrees, palms facing up. Allow body to relax into the earth and breathe deeply and evenly. (If this puts strain on lower back, bend your knees.)

CRADLE ROCK (Apanasana): Draw your knees into your chest and wrap your arms around the upper part of your shins. Gently rock back and forth.

EASY POSE (Sukhasana): With bottom on floor, cross legs in a comfortable position, rest hands on knees, palms facing up for more energy, facing down to bring more relaxation. Lengthen spine by reaching crown towards the sky, open chest to allow for full expansion of lungs.

CAT-COW: Start in table top position, knees under hips, wrists under shoulders, spine neutral. Curl your toes under, inhale and slowly stretch your back, looking up to sky and extending tail bone toward ceiling (cow). Uncurl toes and on the exhale round the lower back (Cat), gently drawing the belly towards the spine. Fluid movement...

DOWNWARD FACING DOG (Adho Mukha Svanasana): Curl toes under and push back, raising hips towards sky and straightening legs. Position hands shoulder width apart, feet hip width apart. Weight is evenly distributed front and back. Lower heels towards floor. Allow your head to gently hang between arms, chest towards earth.

209

MOUNTAIN (Tadasana): Stand erect with feet hip width apart (or if your balance is good you can have feet touching). Hands loose at sides, spine lengthened, shoulders up, back and down, eyes gaze forward. Feel the earth beneath your feet.

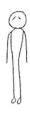

TREE (Vrksasana): Begin in mountain. Bring your weight onto your left foot, feeling the earth, coming into balance. Place the sole of your right foot on the inside of your left thigh (or calf or ankle - but NOT on knee). Bring hands into prayer pose at heart (or raise above head, palms together.) Repeat opposite side.

FORWARD BEND (Uttanasana): Start in mountain. Take hands up to sky, then exhale, bend at the waist, sweeping arms down. Legs can be straight or knees slightly bent if hams feel stiff. Keep weight toward the front of your feet to avoid leaning backwards. Relax your neck, allowing the crown of your head to reach toward the ground.

EXTENDED CHILD / FULL CHILD: Sit on your feet, knees comfortably separated, straighten your back and lift up, stretch arms out in front of you and relax your neck, resting head between arms. For full child, wrap your arms around your body, palms facing up by feet. Remember to breathe!

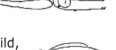

THUNDERBOLT (Vajrasana): Sit back on your calves, take care that your chest is open and your spine is long and straight. Balance head and neck over pelvic region. Allow hands to rest on thighs.

STAFF POSE (Dandasana): Sit with your legs stretched out in front of you, legs touching and parallel to the floor. Sit up straight. Place hands next to hip area, spine long, thigh muscles engaged, heels slightly lifted off floor. Contract abs, open shoulders, elongate spine, crown towards ceiling and gaze gently forward.

Root Chakra - Earth Meditation

Become mindful of the moment: Be aware of where you find yourself NOW. The past is a memory... the future only a whisper of what might be. What exists between them is this present moment. Observe this interlude, this synapse in time and rest there.

Become mindful of your body... the weight being supported by the floor, the beating of your heart, the breath flowing, inhaling and exhaling the earth breath, in and out through your nose. Feel it flow into your being, filling your lungs to capacity. Even and full. Even and full.

Now bring that mindfulness to your feelings. What sensations are you experiencing in your body? Are there areas of tension or rigidity? Breathe into them... Allow them to relax. As you fully exhale, let them flow out of your being, at the same time, expressing gratitude that your body is sharing a message with you.

If stray thoughts enter your mind, gently let them float by like wisps of a cloud and bring your attention back to this present moment and your breath.

Now bring your awareness back to the weight of your body. Feel the effects of gravity as it gets heavier ... tension, stress, negative energies melting and dissipating. Guide your intention to the soles of your feet. Picture a light that extends out from the feet and down through the floor into the ground. Allow it to merge with the magnetic core center of Mother Earth. This light bonds with her love and establishes a gentle rootedness. Continue to breathe evenly and fully, almost as if your breath is now breathing you.

With every inhale this wonderful earth energy and light rise up - up - up through every part of your physical body, illuminating all of your cells, every fiber of your being, until it reaches your crown...

Then it begins its return journey, flowing back down towards the earth, a continuous, infinite stream of vitality as you inhale and exhale. Even and full.

This 'cord' of light and breath is your anchor. Moment by moment, whatever is transpiring in your life, know that you are linked to the earth, thus allowing your heart and your mind and your spirit to soar while you remain connected and grounded.

Like a tree with roots firmly entrenched in the earth, but whose branches are free to sway and bend and flow with the wind, you are a beautiful blend of rootedness and flexibility.

Now allow your breath to rest in Muladhara, the root chakra, in a beautiful warm red light glowing at the base of your spine. Affirm to yourself: I am lovingly guided, lovingly protected and all of my needs are met.

Continue to breathe gently and easily now. Balanced, anchored and energized.

You are home.

ENERGY TYPES

Sacral Chakra Toolkit

Location: Sacral/Pelvic Region
Related Color: Orange

When BALANCED... We are able to 'go with the flow,' feeling comfortable with change as we ride the tide of life.

We feel motivated to act on our passion and desires, cultivating our relationship to self and to others in our lives.

When the SCALES ARE TIPPED...

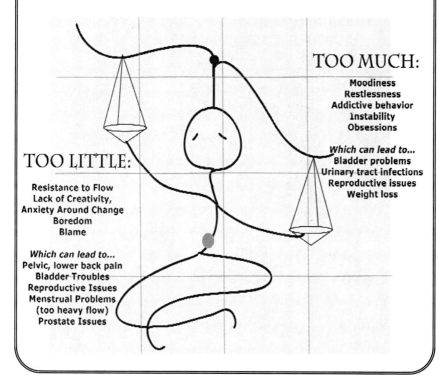

TOO MUCH:

Moodiness
Restlessness
Addictive behavior
Instability
Obsessions

Which can lead to...
Bladder problems
Urinary tract infections
Reproductive issues
Weight loss

TOO LITTLE:

Resistance to Flow
Lack of Creativity,
Anxiety Around Change
Boredom
Blame

Which can lead to...
Pelvic, lower back pain
Bladder Troubles
Reproductive Issues
Menstrual Problems
(too heavy flow)
Prostate Issues

refreshed and free

snow-capped white mountains
usher melting Spring falls
cascading in streams
blending in rivers
and merging with oceans
of our souls...
alight with movement, passion
and becoming...
transforming the seasons of our lives
as newness settles into the very cells
of our being -
cleansed now,
refreshed and free.

- *Maureen*

SACRAL CHAKRA - SVADISTHANA ("ONE'S OWN PLACE")

*T*he sacral chakra, our second energy field, is located in the pelvic region of our body and corresponds most specifically to the process of creation, to relationships and flow. If our root chakra, linked with the element of the earth, is providing a strong foundation, then the sacral chakra will be 'ripe' for planting.

Associated with the element of water, it provides the fertility for what we produce in our lives, both from an actual place of sexuality as well as motivation behind ideas and their manifestation. Water, fluid and formless, simultaneously purifies and nourishes. Depending upon our constitution, our bodies are generally made up of between 70% and 90% water. As this beautiful element is the conductor of life energy (prana), the importance of flow in our lives cannot be understated.

With our sacral chakra in balance, we feel motivated and ready to try new things. This energy field is associated with the color of orange.

Here are some questions to ask yourself to determine your balance in the SACRAL CHAKRA:

You may be Sacral Chakra deficient if you answer 'yes'
to any of the following:

* *Am I feeling bored with my life and ready to seek out new experiences and opportunities?*
* *Am I expressing my needs and desires but not taking action to support them?*

217

* *Does my level of creativity feel like it could use an infusion of new energy?*
* *Am I being resistant to the flow of my life?*

If you responded positively to any of these questions, you might want to visit the SACRAL CHAKRA TOOLKIT. Our second chakra is all about movement and flow. Expression is wonderful but we need to 'walk our talk.' Bring your ideas into action!

You may be in Sacral Chakra excess if you answer 'yes' to any of the following:

* *Am I feeling energized and but restless and without direction?*
* *Am I having a difficult time expressing what it is I am passionate about?*
* *Am I obsessing over people or things causing unhealthy expenditures of energy?*
* *Are my moods interfering with the process of manifesting?*

If you responded in the affirmative to any of *these* questions, chances are you need to spend some time either establishing ROOTS in the FIRST CHAKRA TOOLKIT or embracing your own truth with the THROAT CHAKRA TOOLKIT. This is the seat of self-expression. By sharing your visions as well as taking an authentic look inside yourself for guidance, you may find the clarity you need as well as assistance in bringing your endeavors to reality.

Sacral Chakra: Breathwork & Mudras

WATER BREATH: Inhale through the nose, picturing a blue-green cascading waterfall entering through the crown, flowing down and filling your heart space. As you then exhale through the mouth, see the water pouring out in a fine stream through your hands, feet, and spine washing away any tension, anxiety or pain. As you release what is not serving you, this energy pours into the ground where Mother Earth welcomes it, transmutes it, and uses this energy to aid her in the rejuvenation of any areas where she is needing healing and sustenance.

USHAS MUDRA (BREAK OF DAY/DAWN): Clasp hands and rest in front of lower belly. Males place right thumb on top of left, females place left thumb on top of right. (Gertrud Hirschi - Mudras: Yoga In Your Hands[1]) This mudra inspires creativity, like the planting of seeds in fertile ground.

BHUDI MUDRA (FLUID MUDRA): Bring tips of thumb and little finger together, others extended. This 'hand yoga' position is important for restoration or maintainence of the fluid balance in our body.

Sacral Chakra Intention:

Working with the sacral chakra flow will allow you to bring movement and energy to the creative desires within you. Here you take the stability and foundation of the root chakra and through breath and movement, nurture the fertile earth with the seeds of intention and motivation.

Affirmation for Sacral Chakra:

I flow easily and fluidly with the current of my life.
I am the river.

SACRAL CHAKRA FLOW

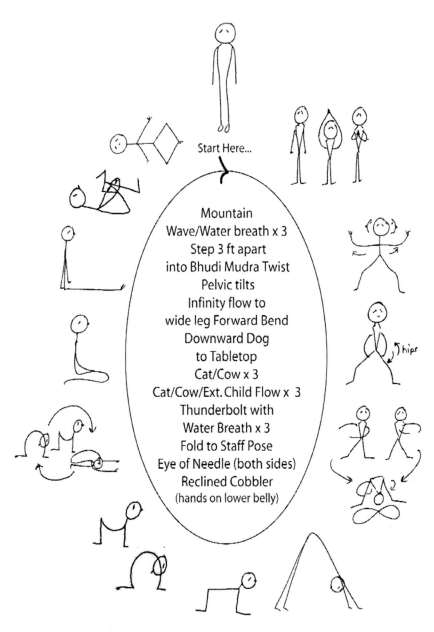

Start Here...

Mountain
Wave/Water breath x 3
Step 3 ft apart
into Bhudi Mudra Twist
Pelvic tilts
Infinity flow to
wide leg Forward Bend
Downward Dog
to Tabletop
Cat/Cow x 3
Cat/Cow/Ext. Child Flow x 3
Thunderbolt with
Water Breath x 3
Fold to Staff Pose
Eye of Needle (both sides)
Reclined Cobbler
(hands on lower belly)

Description of YOGA POSES for **Sacral Chakra Flow:**

As with all poses listed here in Energy Types, please modify to suit your own particular strength, flexibility and/or health challenges.

MOUNTAIN (Tadasana): Stand erect with feet hip width apart (or if your balance is good you can have feet touching). Hands loose at sides, spine lengthened, shoulders up, back and down, eyes gaze forward. Feel the earth beneath your feet.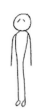

WAVE WATER BREATH: Come into water breath, inhaling through the nose and exhaling through the mouth. On your inhale, take the arms out to the sides and up overhead, bringing palms together, and as you exhale, bringing hands down to the chest, prayer hands at heart in Anjali Mudra. (Repeat this three times.)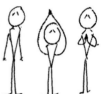

BHUDI MUDRA TWIST Bring the breath to a natural flow just through the nose and step your feet into a wider stance, perhaps 2 to 2 1/2 feet apart. Bring a slight bend to the knees. Take the arms up to the sky and out to the sides, palms up and come into Bhudi Mudra, thumb and pinky finger together. As you exert slight pressure between the fingers, gently turn the body from side to side, into Bhudi Mudra twist.
Continue this movement back and forth about 6 times and then come back to face center.

PELVIC TILTS: Take the hands down to your hips and gently come into a few pelvic tilts. Inhale, taking shoulders and bottom back, slight arch, and as you exhale, round the back and tilt the pelvis forward. Repeat 3 or 4 times with your breath, activating the sacral chakra.

INFINITY FLOW: Keeping the feet the same distance apart, straighten the legs and begin to flow the arms in a figure 8 motion from side to side, right to left, left to right, bending the knee on either side as the arms flow over that side. Keep breathing nice full breaths, totally letting your arms joyfully swing to and fro... and then start to take this motion into a fold, ending in a wide-legged forward bend.

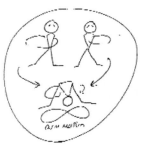

DOWNWARD FACING DOG (Adho Mukha Svanasana): Curl toes under and push back, raising hips towards sky and straightening legs. Position hands shoulder width apart, feet hip width apart. Weight is evenly distributed front and back. Lower heels towards floor. Allow your head to gently hang between arms, chest towards earth.

CAT-COW: Start in table top position, knees under hips, wrists under shoulders, spine neutral. Curl your toes under, inhale and slowly stretch your back, looking up to sky and extending tail bone toward ceiling (cow). Uncurl toes and on the exhale round the lower back (Cat), gently drawing the belly towards the spine. Fluid movement...

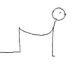

CAT-COW FLOW: Inhale, looking up, then exhale, arch and push your bottom back into extended child, bend your elbows and glide your chest along the floor inhaling once more back up to cow pose. Repeat this sequence, exhaling, arch and push bottom back to extended child, inhale glide up to cow...

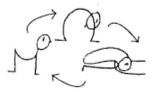

THUNDERBOLT (Vajrasana): Sit back on your calves, take care that your chest is open and your spine is long and straight. Balance head and neck over pelvic region. Allow hands to rest on thighs.

STAFF POSE (Dandasana): Sit with your legs stretched out in front of you, legs touching and parallel to the floor. Sit up straight. Place hands next to hip area, spine long, thigh muscles engaged, heels slightly lifted off floor. Contract abs, open shoulders, elongate spine, crown towards ceiling and gaze gently forward.

EYE OF THE NEEDLE (Sucirandhrasana): From prone postition, place both feet next to your bottom, flat on the earth. Draw your right leg in and cross the right ankle over the left knee. Stretch your right hand through the v-shaped hole this forms and clasp hands behind the left thigh. Use your right elbow to push against the right thigh, further enhancing the stretch in the hip area. Repeat on opposite side.

RECLINED COBBLER (Supta Badha Konasana):   Lie flat, feet flat on floor next to bottom, lower knees away from each other and bring soles of feet together. Elongate neck area by bringing shoulders down from ears. Hands rest alongside body, palms facing up.

Sacral Chakra Meditation

Take a moment to bring yourself into the present, tuning into your internal clock that ticks gently to the sound of your heartbeat, and close your eyes. Relax your jaw, your shoulders, all of your muscles and just be. Begin to practice the Water Breath, bringing your inhale in through the nose, and exhaling gently and fully through the mouth. With every breath, you release any tension, any worries... just let them go. In through the nose, out through the mouth. A sigh of surrender, bringing to mind our intention for Svadisthana... embracing and allowing the exquisite waves of creation that exist within you to emerge unimpeded.

Now as you continue to ride the tide of your inhale and exhale, picture a beautiful river flowing through you. The river of your breath... the river of your blood... the river of the energy coursing through you.... and become this river.

Affirm the following...

I am the river.

I flow easily and fluidly with the current of my life.

I am the river.

I release my fingers from the banks and let the momentum carry me...

I am the river.

I flow over and around all perceived obstacles and rocks in my path.. knowing my course is true.

I am the river.

The pace of my flow is guided by an internal knowing...
sometimes rapid, sometimes slow and gentle.

I am the river.

My allowance of flow leads me to the source...
to an ocean of unlimited love, joy, abundance and potential.

I am the river.

Relax now into this lovely space you have created within you, a place of serenity and calm. In the flow. You are the river.

Solar Plexus Chakra Toolkit

Location: Solar Plexus Region
Related Color: Yellow

When BALANCED...

Our sense of self-esteem is firmly intact and our 'warrior' qualities shine like the sun.

We move forward in our lives with confidence and purpose.

When the SCALES ARE TIPPED...

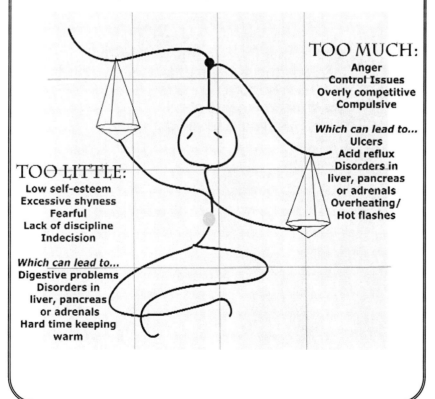

TOO MUCH:
Anger
Control Issues
Overly competitive
Compulsive

Which can lead to...
Ulcers
Acid reflux
Disorders in
liver, pancreas
or adrenals
Overheating/
Hot flashes

TOO LITTLE:
Low self-esteem
Excessive shyness
Fearful
Lack of discipline
Indecision

Which can lead to...
Digestive problems
Disorders in
liver, pancreas
or adrenals
Hard time keeping
warm

awaiting the 'great' revelation
when, maybe, the 'revealing'
is truly nothing more
than a peeling back of the shroud
preventing light
from shining through.
release fear and
pull back the curtains.
bask in the always present glow.
and in that light you may learn that
perhaps the 'a-ha' moment
we seek is that there are
no 'a-ha' moments at all.
ever changing.   never changing.
'a-ha.'
(or not.)

- *Maureen*

SOLAR PLEXUS CHAKRA
MANIPURA ("LUSTROUS GEM")

*T*he solar plexus chakra, our third energy field, is located in the abdominal area and represents our center of self-esteem. This is the relationship we have with ourselves and where we claim our personal power and confidence. It is associated with the color of vibrant yellow and by picturing this beautiful sun shining within us, we can greatly enhance the energy that Manipura so awesomely bestows.

The solar plexus is represented by the element of fire and provides 'filtration through burning' i.e. removal of what is no longer serving us through the process of 'burning it out.'

Applying the grounding of the root chakra and the movement and desire offered by our balanced sacral chakra, "Manipura" contributes the warmth and sunlight needed to give those seeds of manifestation the 'oomph' they need to grow and thrive! The heat provided by the solar plexus chakra also has a direct correlation with our metabolism, digestion and transformation of our food into energy. The major organs associated with these processes are also affected by this chakra and can therefore manifest as associated physical ailments.

Following are questions to ask yourself to determine your balance in the SOLAR PLEXUS CHAKRA:

You may be Solar Plexus Chakra deficient if you answer 'yes' to any of the following:

* *Am I lacking the strength to make an important life decision?*
* *Do I procrastinate around taking charge of my life out of fear?*

229

* *Am I a sponge for other people's pain, so much so that I can't absorb anything more?*
* *Am I allowing the opinions of others to derail my own personal needs or desires?*

If you responded positively to any of these questions, it may be time to visit the SOLAR PLEXUS CHAKRA TOOLKIT and your center of self-esteem. Building your core strength will allow you to say 'no' to those situations that are depleting you and very possibly leading to the enabling of others. (Compassionate detachment is a lesson that many overly-empathic folks may need to learn.) The more we shine inside ourselves, the brighter our example.

You may be in Solar Plexus Chakra excess if you answer 'yes' to any of the following:

* *Am I feeling prone to anger in my everyday life?*
* *Am I finding that I am overly competitive?*
* *Do I find myself having a hard time accepting the love of others?*

If you answered in the affirmative to any of *these* questions, chances are you may need to spend some time either practicing self-care with the HEART CHAKRA TOOLKIT or 'cooling down' with the SACRAL CHAKRA TOOLKIT. In order to truly honor our personal power, we need to come from a healthy sense of self-confidence. Fire is a mighty tool, but dangerous when out of control.

Solar Plexus Chakra: Breathwork & Mudras

FIRE BREATH: Become aware of the beating of your heart and the brilliant sun inside your core. Bring the awareness to the breath flowing evenly in and out of your nose. Now start to inhale through the mouth, sipping the air in and directing it into the radiance of your solar plexus chakra, the sun within you, allowing the light to expand and rise up to fill your heart space. Exhale through the nose and send this light out into the space in front of you, on to your path of purpose. Continue this flow, inhaling through the mouth, exhaling through the nose...

RUDRA MUDRA: (Ruler of the Solar Plexus) Bring thumb, index finger and ring finger together. Extend other two fingers in a relaxed manner. This will combat weakness.

MATANGI MUDRA: (Matangi - God of Inner Harmony) Clasp hands in front of solar plexus, with only middle fingers extending upwards, resting against one another. This mudra will improve the breathwork in this area of the body, increase energy and enthusiasm, as well as aid digestion.

> ### Solar Plexus Chakra Intention:
> Working with the solar plexus flow will 'stoke the fire' within you, energizing you and rekindling feelings of confidence and inner power.
>
> ### Affirmation for Solar Plexus Chakra:
> I claim my personal power and move forward with confidence and courage. I embrace the light and fire of the the sun within me.

SOLAR PLEXUS CHAKRA FLOW

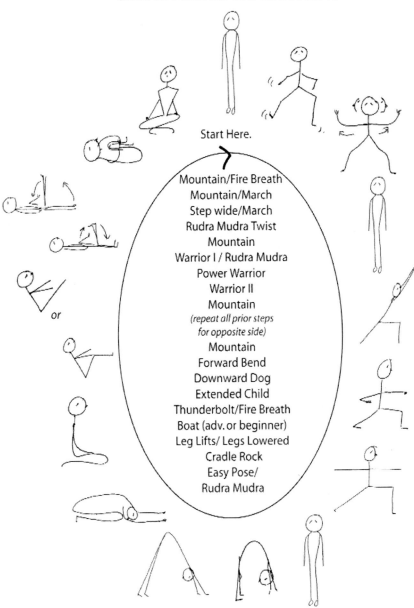

Start Here.

Mountain/Fire Breath
Mountain/March
Step wide/March
Rudra Mudra Twist
Mountain
Warrior I / Rudra Mudra
Power Warrior
Warrior II
Mountain
*(repeat all prior steps
for opposite side)*
Mountain
Forward Bend
Downward Dog
Extended Child
Thunderbolt/Fire Breath
Boat (adv. or beginner)
Leg Lifts/ Legs Lowered
Cradle Rock
Easy Pose/
Rudra Mudra

or

Description of YOGA POSES for
Solar Plexus Chakra Flow:

As with all poses listed here in Energy Types, please modify to suit your own particular strength, flexibility and/or health challenges.

MOUNTAIN (Tadasana): Stand erect with feet hip width apart (or if your balance is good you can have feet touching). Hands loose at sides, spine lengthened, shoulders up, back and down, eyes gaze forward. Feel the earth beneath your feet. Begin practicing the fire breath, in through the mouth, out through the nose.

MARCH: Now bring your breath back to an easy inhale and exhale just through the nose and begin to march, feet drawing earth energy up into your being and activating your inner power. As you become one with the motion, feel the blood flowin and your heart beating. Now step just a little wider, feet 2 -1/2 to 3 feet apart, and continue to march, swinging the arms in rhythm with your movement, further enhancing the energy flow within you.

RUDRA MUDRA TWIST Keeping your wide stance, ground the feet and sweep you arms first up over head and out to your sides in 'Rudra Mudra' - the ruler of the solar plexus chakra - by bringing the tips of thumb, index and ring fingers together. Gently begin to twist from side to side, continuing to breathe deep, expansive breaths. Make sure that you are fully exhaling to allow fresh new air to flow back in.

233

WARRIOR I (Virabhadrasana I): Step your right foot back and ground it at a 45 degree angle, left foot also grounded and knee directly over ankle bent to 90 degrees. Bringing hands into rudra mudra, extend them up towards the sky and glance up as well towards the sun. Hold for 3 breaths before moving into...

POWER WARRIOR: Lower arms to waist level, create fists with hands, thumb encircled by other fingers, and draw right arm back, fist adjacent to side ribs, elbow pointing behind you. Again hold posture for 3 breaths.

WARRIOR II (Virabhadrasana II): Release fists, sweep right arm in a forward circle, and back behind you, back foot now at 90 degrees, arms parallel to earth, straight line from sternum to pelvis, and gaze out over extended left arm. Hold 3 breaths.

FORWARD BEND (Uttanasana): Start in mountain. Take hands up to sky, then exhale, bend at the waist, sweeping arms down. Legs can be straight or knees slightly bent if hams feel stiff. Keep weight toward the front of your feet to avoid leaning backwards. Relax your neck, allowing the crown of your head to reach toward the ground.

DOWNWARD FACING DOG (Adho Mukha Svanasana): Curl toes under and push back, raising hips towards sky and straightening legs. Position hands shoulder width apart, feet hip width apart. Weight is evenly distributed front and back. Lower heels towards floor. Allow your head to gently hang between arms, chest towards earth.

EXTENDED CHILD: Sit on your feet, knees comfortably separated, straighten your back and lift up, stretch arms out in front of you and relax your neck, resting head between arms.

THUNDERBOLT (Vajrasana): Sit back on your calves, take care that your chest is open and your spine is long and straight. Balance head and neck over pelvic region. Allow hands to rest on thighs.

BOAT POSE (Navasana): Fold over and stretch legs out in front of you. Depending on your ability to balance and strength of your abs, first ground hands on either side of hips and bend knees, lifting legs so that calves are parallel to earth. You can hold here, or draw arms up, palms facing one another - hold here OR straighten legs, keeping spine long and straight.

LEG LIFTS: Lower all the way down to the floor, stretching arms and legs out on mat. Now place your hands palms down underneath your bottom to protect your lower back. Draw knees into your chest on an inhale, and exhale, kick the legs out in front of you, toes pointed, inhale lift to sky and draw knees back into chest. Repeat 5 times. Then with knees into chest, inhale, kick feet up to sky, feet flexed, on exhale, lower heels slowly towards the earth (not quite touching) and then inhale knees back to chest. Repeat 5 times again ending with knees into chest.

CRADLE ROCK (Apanasana):Draw your knees into your chest and wrap your arms around the upper part of your shins. Gently rock back and forth.

EASY POSE (Sukhasana): With bottom on floor, cross legs in a comfortable position, rest hands on knees, palms facing up for more energy, facing down to bring more relaxation. Lengthen spine by reaching crown towards the sky, open chest to allow for full expansion of lungs. (Hands can also be placed on knees in rudra mudra.)

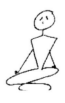

Solar Plexus Chakra Flow Cave Fire Meditation

Close your eyes and come to a quiet place in your mind... Allow outside thoughts and distractions to become more and more distant. Begin breathing the fire breath: Inhaling long, fresh breaths through your mouth, sipping air, and exhaling gently through the nose, bringing a sense of calm to your being. Use the rhythm of the breath as an anchor. Keep your attention there until the mind relaxes and becomes serene. Now draw your awareness to any life situation that may be challenging you or any dream you are aching to fulfill. Allow this intention to rest in your core as you continue to breathe evenly and fully.

See yourself walking along a path that leads to the entrance of a cave. You proceed down a series of steps, one at a time to the quiet, cool inner expanse of the cavern. As you adjust to the initial darkness, your eyes are drawn to a fire pit glowing in the center of the chamber. Beautiful orange and gold flames are illuminating the cave and casting long shadows on the black walls...

You are drawn now to the hearth and settle down directly in front of it, feeling the intense heat on your hands, on your face... You hear the crackling of the logs as the sap hits the fire.

As you stare into the flames, repeat your intention. What question do you need answered? What decision needs to be made? What goal are you longing to fulfill? What needs to be released?

Bring your attention to the flames. Become one with the dancing, flickering fire. Feel the heat, the passion, the fire within your own core. You radiate this same energy. Know with all of your being that as you become absolutely clear about specific goals and intentions in your life, you will step up with passion and power to take whatever action is necessary to achieve your desired results.

Keep breathing now... long, calm breaths. In through the mouth, out through the nose. Trust the personal power in your third chakra... Manipura... your solar plexus.

Know you have ignited a fire of focus within you, committed now to bringing these internal images into being. *Affirm in true knowing,* "I claim my inner power and move forward with confidence and courage. I embrace the light and fire of the the sun within me."

All is well.

Heart Chakra Toolkit

Location: Heart/Chest Region
Related Color: Green

When BALANCED...

Compassion flows easily out from our heart as well as back into our heart... A circle of love.

We sense our connection to all other beings and find peace in this unity.

When the SCALES ARE TIPPED...

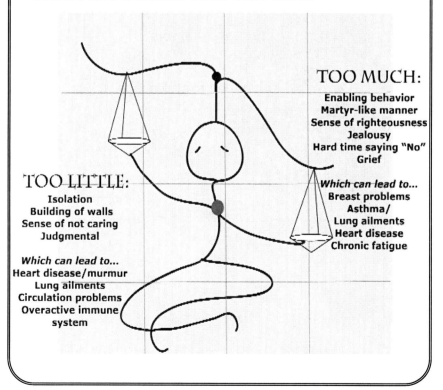

TOO MUCH:
Enabling behavior
Martyr-like manner
Sense of righteousness
Jealousy
Hard time saying "No"
Grief

Which can lead to...
Breast problems
Asthma/
Lung ailments
Heart disease
Chronic fatigue

TOO LITTLE:
Isolation
Building of walls
Sense of not caring
Judgmental

Which can lead to...
Heart disease/murmur
Lung ailments
Circulation problems
Overactive immune system

Dear God,
Allow me to create boundaries
but not armor...
to be compassionate
without losing myself...
to understand my role of teacher
if need be
by educating through example
and not rescuing...
and finally,
allow me to surrender to the process
knowing your sweet angels
are doing the same
for me.

- *Maureen*

HEART CHAKRA
ANAHATA ("UNSTRUCK")

*O*ur remarkable heart chakra resides in the center of our energy fields, bridging the physical and spiritual realms. I consider the this chakra to be the 'captain of our ship,' bringing earth, water and fire into conjunction with sound, light and the Divine. And while all of our chakras are interrelated, the heart is the realm that provides the authenticity of any thought, action or intention flowing through any other field. Being 'true to our heart' is the kindest, healthiest endeavor we can undertake.

'Anahata' is the seat of compassion and associated with the element of air. By bringing increased awareness to the gift of our breath, we experience "inspiration" in the true sense of the word, as we fill our lungs and being with fresh, vital life force. Our exhale becomes a heart-felt bond with all sentient beings, united through our breath. When we realize this connection, we also begin to understand the importance of monitoring our thoughts and intentions, as this energy penetrates our very environment and personal domain in so many ways. Of particular note when considering the magnanimous qualities of our heart is the following statistic from the Institute of Hearth Math: *"The magnetic field produced by the heart is more than 5,000 times greater in strength than the field generated by the brain, and can be detected a number of feet away from the body, in all directions."* [2]

To achieve true balance within our hearts, we must practice both giving as well as receiving. "Self love is not selfish. It is self esteem," as author Melody Beattie so eloquently states in her book, *The Language of Letting Go.*[3] Allow love to fill your heart with compassion first for

241

yourself and then the love you share with others will come from a place of authenticity. In traditional Yogic philosophy, the heart chakra is represented by the color of emerald green.

Below are questions to ask yourself to determine your balance in the HEART CHAKRA:

You may be Heart Chakra deficient if you answer 'yes' to any of the following:

* *Am I finding it difficult to accept love?*
* *Have I erected a wall around myself to avoid getting hurt?*
* *Am I finding it difficult to forgive?*
* *Have I lost my sense of connection with others in my life?*

If you answered positively to any of these questions, it may be time to visit the HEART CHAKRA TOOLKIT and open the channels of love.

You may be in Heart Chakra excess if you answer 'yes' to any of the following:

* *Have I given so much of myself that there is nothing left to give?*
* *Do I feel jealousy when I see others acting carefree and joyful?*
* *Am I going through a grieving process or time of loss?*
* *Do I have a hard time saying "No?"*

If you answered in the affirmative to any of *these* questions, you may need to recharge your sense of self-esteem and personal power with the SOLAR PLEXUS TOOLKIT or reestablish the 'ground rules' and reconnect to your right to have, to be and TO BE LOVED with the ROOT CHAKRA TOOLKIT. Once feeling grounded and 'courageous' (the root of this word being HEART), return to the HEART CHAKRA TOOLKIT to replenish your center of love.

Heart Chakra: Breathwork & Mudras

HEART BREATH: As you come into a quiet place within you, allowing each moment to gently unfold, direct your awareness into the beautiful chamber of your heart. Become one with your pulse and the life flowing through you. As your attention rests peacefully in this center of love, allow the breath and the heartbeat to become synchronized, in a beautiful current of rhythm, breathing in and out for the same number of beats. After establishing a comfortable pattern, begin to bring the inhale in through the left side of the heart, receiving love, letting it fill your being. Then send the exhale out through the right side of the heart, giving love back. Continue to allow your breath to form a circle of love around you, the compassion and gift of giving and receiving, radiating out into ever-widening circles of light and radiance... Giving and receiving... Loving balance, all encompassing, reaching to the ends of the Universe.

AIR BREATH: The heart chakra is represented by the element of air. In the 'air breath,' we inhale and exhale out of the mouth in a gentle, smooth circle of flow, deepening our concept of unity consciousness, becoming one with the breath of the Universe. The focus will also be on the expansion of the heart space.

** *For more information on similar patterns of breathwork and meditation, I highly recommend the practice of HEART RHYTHM MEDITATION with Puran & Susanna Bair. Learn more at www.iamheart.org.*[4]

PADME MUDRA (LOTUS MUDRA): Bring the heels of the palms together, touch thumbs and little fingers, all other fingers pointing upwards like the blossoming of a lotus. Hold gently on heart space.

CHIN MUDRA: (UNITY CONSCIOUSNESS) Bring thumb and index fingers together, all other fingers extended. The index finger correlates with the heart chakra, and this mudra also represents the inter-connectedness of all life.

Heart Chakra Intention:
Allowing ourselves to not only give love, but to also be receptive of love, as we learn that we cannot serve others from an empty well. Practice a Universal Love Exchange...

Affirmation for Heart Chakra:
I give and receive love with ease and celebrate my connection and compassion with all sentient beings.

HEART CHAKRA FLOW

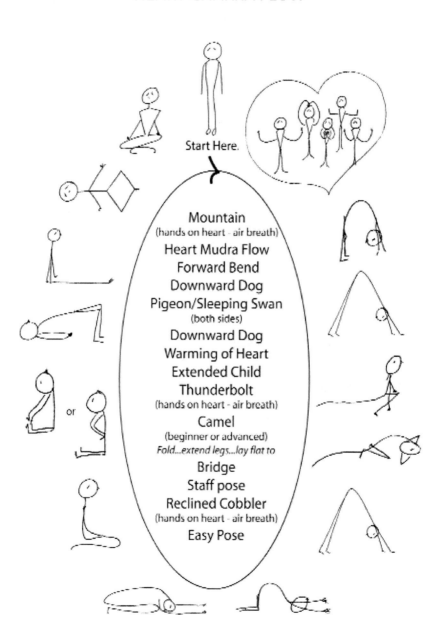

Start Here.

Mountain
(hands on heart - air breath)
Heart Mudra Flow
Forward Bend
Downward Dog
Pigeon/Sleeping Swan
(both sides)
Downward Dog
Warming of Heart
Extended Child
Thunderbolt
(hands on heart - air breath)
Camel
(beginner or advanced)
Fold....extend legs...lay flat to
Bridge
Staff pose
Reclined Cobbler
(hands on heart - air breath)
Easy Pose

or

Description of YOGA POSES for
Heart Chakra Flow:

As with all poses listed here in Energy Types, please modify to suit your own particular strength, flexibility and/or health challenges.

MOUNTAIN (Tadasana): Stand erect with feet hip width apart (or if your balance is good you can have feet touching). Hands loose at sides, spine lengthened, shoulders up, back and down, eyes gaze forward. Feel the earth beneath your feet.

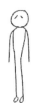

HEART MUDRA FLOW: Take arms out to sides, fingers in Chin Mudra (thumb and index finger joined), palms up, bent elbows. Inhale, raising hands up to sky , then resting fingertips on crown. Lower hands as you exhale, palms facing you, down to heart level, then push them out in front of you and sweep open to sides, palms still facing outward in a gesture of spreading heart radiance into the space around you, then back to chin mudra, hands out to sides. Repeat 4 times in honor of 4th Chakra.

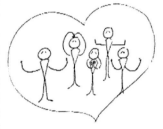

FORWARD BEND (Uttanasana): Start in mountain. Take hands up to sky, then exhale, bend at the waist, sweeping arms down. Legs can be straight or knees slightly bent if hams feel stiff. Keep weight toward the front of your feet to avoid leaning backwards. Relax your neck, allowing the crown of your head to reach toward the ground.

DOWNWARD FACING DOG (Adho Mukha Svanasana): Curl toes under and push back, raising hips towards sky and straightening legs. Position hands shoulder width apart, feet hip width apart. Weight evenly distributed front and back. Lower heels towards floor. Allow your head to gently hang between arms, chest towards earth.

PIGEON/SLEEPING SWAN: From down dog, draw right knee between hands, lean over to right hip, stretching left leg out, open chest area by broadening shoulders, rising up on finger tips. Come into sleeping swan by gently crossing arms in front of you and lowering head to forearms. Rest here for a few breaths before easing back up to pigeon. Repeat opposite side.

WARMING OF HEART (Anahatasana): Also called "puppy dog." From table top (or down dog), hips over knees, extend arms forward, forehead moves towards floor, hips toward sky, and heart melts towards the earth. If shoulders feel constricted, move arms wider apart.

EXTENDED CHILD: Sit on your feet, knees comfortably separated, straighten your back and lift up, stretch arms out in front of you and relax your neck, resting head between arms.

THUNDERBOLT (Vajrasana): Sit back on your calves, take care that your chest is open and your spine is long and straight. Balance head and neck over pelvic region. Allow hands to rest on thighs.

CAMEL (Utrasana): Beginners: Rise up to knees, bring hands, fingertips pointing up, to lower back and gently lean back, looking up at ceiling. More advanced, reach hands to heels. In either case, feel expansion of chest area.

247

BRIDGE (Setu Bandhasana): Lie on mat, bend knees & place feet flat on floor directly over ankles. Let weight of hips and back of shoulders sink into floor and draw shoulders down from ears. Point chin towards chest. Press into feet and lift hips off mat. Either press hands into floor next to hip area or clasp hands under bottom, further expanding heart space. To come out, remove hands and gently lower spine to floor.

STAFF POSE (Dandasana): Sit with legs stretched out in front of you, parallel to floor. Sit up straight. Place hands next to hip area, spine long, thigh muscles engaged, heels slightly lifted off floor. Contract abs, open shoulders, elongate spine, crown towards ceiling & gaze forward.

RECLINED COBBLER (Supta Badha Konasana):   Lie flat, feet flat on floor next to bottom, lower knees away from each other and bring soles of feet together. Elongate neck area by bringing shoulders down from ears. Hands rest alongside body, palms facing up.

EASY POSE (Sukhasana): With bottom on floor, cross legs in a comfortable position, rest hands on knees, palms facing up for more energy, facing down to bring more relaxation. Lengthen spine by reaching crown towards the sky, open chest to allow for full expansion of lungs.

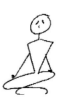

248

Heart Chakra Meditation

Now is your time. Allow any outside distractions to just fade away as you close your eyes and come home to yourself, this beautiful chamber deep inside your heart. As your awareness gently rests here in this sacred space, breathe and allow the love within you to expand and glow. Become one with your heart beat... sense the pulse, the life flowing through you, your connection to the world.

See if you can bring your breath and your heartbeat into coherence... a matching pattern of lifeforce, breathing to the rhythm within you... the beat of your inner drum. Constant. Life-giving. Compassion.

With your awareness still keenly on the breath, begin drawing your inhale into the left side of your heart into this receptive chamber, allowing love to flow inside you. Deeply, fully receptive. And as you exhale, send the breath out through the right side of your heart, giving back. Begin forming a circle of radiance around you with your breath, a golden path of light, as you inhale left and exhale right. Inhale left, exhale right. Giving and receiving... Radiating love. Continue with this pattern for the next few breaths... the emerald green in side your heart becoming ever brighter and luminscent.

Now, bring to mind someone to whom you might be sending love, perhaps in need of your prayers, or anyone with whom you might be currently facing a personal challenge. See if you can picture this person seated directly before you... and as you exhale now out the right side of your heart, send your love into the heart of this person, pure compassion entering their being. And as you inhale, you draw their love back into your own. Keep this gentle circle of love flowing for

249

the next few breaths. Giving and receiving...giving and receiving.

Now allow the breath to center itself once more in your own heart chamber. The light within you continues to glow ever brighter on your inhale and with every exhale, flows out into a concentric cir-cle of radiance around you, creating ever-widening ripples of love...

You rest now in the peace of recognizing your universal connection to all sentient beings...merging with the light and radiance of life itself.

Namasté.

Throat Chakra Toolkit

Location: Throat Region
Related Color: Blue

When BALANCED...

We speak our truth with wisdom, clarity and love. Communicating in this voice of authenticity, we share our unique creative expression with the world.

When the SCALES ARE TIPPED...

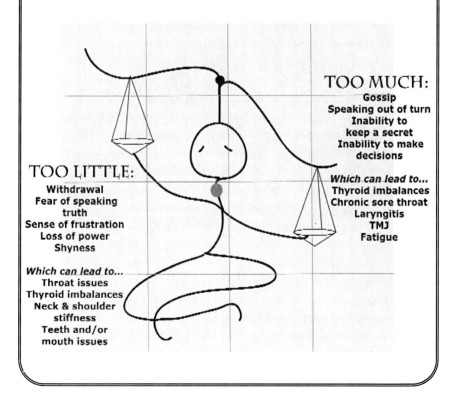

TOO MUCH:
Gossip
Speaking out of turn
Inability to
keep a secret
Inability to make
decisions

Which can lead to...
Thyroid imbalances
Chronic sore throat
Laryngitis
TMJ
Fatigue

TOO LITTLE:
Withdrawal
Fear of speaking
truth
Sense of frustration
Loss of power
Shyness

Which can lead to...
Throat issues
Thyroid imbalances
Neck & shoulder
stiffness
Teeth and/or
mouth issues

without truth what is there?
living life disconnected from the authenticity
of our hearts is participation
in the costliest of facades.

denial of what is...
avoidance of actuality...
leads only to emptiness.

but those 'a-ha' moments,
those glimpses of unfettered joy,
ignite within us the soul-felt belief
in the TRUTH.

though those moments might generally fade,
in their wake remains the knowing.
and in this knowing, the courage to
participate in that dance of authenticity.

invite these awakenings to grace your life
with greater frequency...
and allow the flow of truth to run
uninhibited through your veins.

-Maureen

THROAT CHAKRA
VISSUDHA ("PURIFICATION")

*O*ur 5th energy field, the throat chakra, is the seat of communication and the color of vibrant blue. As every type can experience periods of imbalance that will affect their ability to communicate (both with themselves AND others) this is a key area for all of us to focus some attention. This is the field from which we express ourselves and share our creative gifts with the world and also the narrowest energy field in the body. A bottle-neck can be created when we don't allow ourselves the opportunity to convey thoughts, words or actions that are 'requesting' manifestation.

When suppressed, this stifling of impulse can result in a myriad of consequences including stiffness and pain in upper back, neck and shoulder area. (Hmmm... Think that's where we got the saying, "She/he is a 'pain in the neck?'" Something is not being communicated...) Throat issues, jaw clenching and thyroid imbalances all have their root in the throat chakra. Also of note, the buildup of anger which reflects liver energy/solar plexus 'stuff,' perhaps due to the repercusions of enabling (resentment) or from not feeling heard, can also result in throat chakra imbalances causing effects such as constant throat clearing. Below you will find various combinations of "toolkit flows" to address different issues that can arise around 'Vissudha'.

Following are questions to ask yourself to determine your balance in the THROAT CHAKRA:

You may be Throat Chakra deficient if you answer 'yes' to any of the following:

253

* *Do I find it difficult to express my feelings?*
* *Do I feel I am not being heard (and is this resulting in suppressed feelings of anger or frustration)?*
* *Am I afraid I will hurt someone if I speak my truth?*
* *Do I speak too quickly because I think no one will hear me out?*

If you answered in the positive to any of these questions, it may be time to visit the **THROAT CHAKRA TOOLKIT** and open the channels of communication.

If fear is preventing you from expressing yourself clearly and blocking your creativity, I would suggest doing a **combination flow** that includes **ROOT CHAKRA** (establish a foundation), **SACRAL CHAKRA** (get the current of creation flowing as well as incorporating the cooling element of water) and **THROAT CHAKRA** (once stable and fluid, allow your creative gifts to shine.)

In another scenario, if you feel blocked from speaking your truth because you are afraid of hurting someone, you may want to give the following flow a try: **SOLAR PLEXUS** (fire up your self-esteem), **THROAT CHAKRA** (speak your piece) and **HEART CHAKRA** (allow your compassion to flow in a detached manner.)

You may be in Throat Chakra excess if you answer 'yes' to any of the following:

* *Do I tend to dominate the conversation?*
* *Do I have a hard time keeping a secret?*
* *Am I uncomfortable with silence and chatter unnecessarily to fill any awkward gaps in conversation?*

If you indeed answered "yes" to any of these questions, you may need to reestablish balance in the **THROAT CHAKRA**. If you are feeling overwhelmed with things you would LIKE to express but are having a difficult time due to a lack of direction, here is a flow that can help you find equilibrium. Combine **SACRAL CHAKRA** (cool down any excess fire that may be causing you to 'spout' off and also grease the wheels of creativity), **THIRD EYE** (allow yourself to spend time in quiet contemplation regarding your most beneficial path) and **THROAT CHAKRA** (with awareness on sharing only what is necessary to get your point across and share your gifts).

Throat Chakra: Breathwork & Mudras

UJJAYI BREATH: (Victory Breath) Inhalation and exhalation are both done through the nose. We create an "ocean sound" at the back of the throat by directing the breath there. This can be practiced by first whispering the sound "Ahhhh" with an open mouth as you breathe in and out. Feel the breath caress the back of the throat, like a wave of air. Now, do the same with the mouth closed. The throat passage is narrow, as is the airway, and the breath creates a "rushing" sound. Keep the inhale and exhale of equal length, without strain. It should also bring a calming effect and can actually be used during most any yoga practice.

BEE'S BREATH (Brahmari): This is another form of pranayama that has many benefits such as bringing clarity, focus and calm to the being, but works also very well in massaging the vocal chords. The throat chakra is related to the element of sound and this can bring about healing effects, both physically as well as emotionally. It is taught in a few different manners, but the way I prefer to practice is to place the thumbs over the ears and bring fingertips together at third eye, gently covering the eyes themselves. Then inhale through the nose, and as you exhale, hum. You will feel a mild buzzing within you (sounding much like the drone of a bee). As you allow the gentle humming to foster a sense of overall peace within, consider bringing yourself into communion with the universal vibration of OM.

SHANKH MUDRA (Shell Mudra): Place your left thumb inside the palm of your right hand and close your fingers around it. Raising the fingers of the left hand to point skyward, touch the right thumb to the middle finger of the left hand. Hold your hands in front of you where the heart and throat chakras meet. (This hand position will resemble a conch shell.)

AKASH MUDRA (Space Mudra): Bring tips of thumb and middle fingers together, all others extended. This mudra creates space within us to allow for greater communication and also allows thought and sound to travel more readily by elevating the flow of information between the hemispheres of the brain. It is also said to help alleviate toothaches and reduce ear pain caused by overcongestion.

AND.... **SING!!!** Yep, you heard me. For all of you Extraverts out there, sing in the house, the yard, in line at the bank... Go for it. For you Introverts, close the windows, draw the curtains, turn on the water, and sing your lungs out. It is a great (fun) way to clear the blockages and get the energy flowing. (And don't say "I can't sing." EVERYONE can sing. Ask my 4 cats and 2 dogs, (even though my youngest cat is deaf and maybe *grateful* that he is when

I choose to bellow my own nonsensical tunes throughout the house.) Oh, and by the way, you can add *dancing* to the mix, too. Really get that flow going!

> ## Throat Chakra Intention:
> To allow our self-truth to flow easily and authentically as we communicate both with ourselves and others, thereby unleashing our unique creative gifts in expression to the world.
>
> ## Affirmation for Throat Chakra:
> I speak my truth with wisdom and clarity as I offer my gifts to the world.

THROAT CHAKRA FLOW

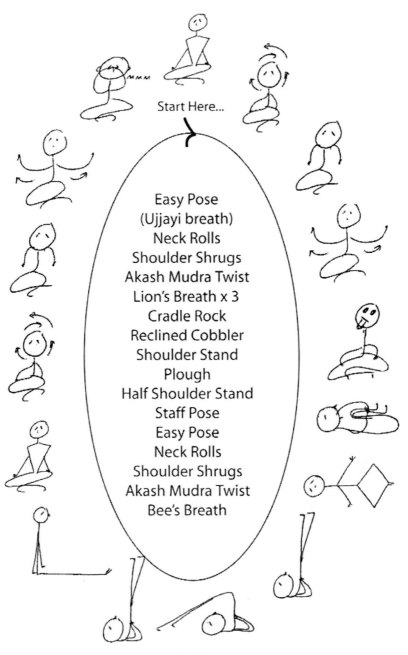

Start Here...

Easy Pose
(Ujjayi breath)
Neck Rolls
Shoulder Shrugs
Akash Mudra Twist
Lion's Breath x 3
Cradle Rock
Reclined Cobbler
Shoulder Stand
Plough
Half Shoulder Stand
Staff Pose
Easy Pose
Neck Rolls
Shoulder Shrugs
Akash Mudra Twist
Bee's Breath

Description of YOGA POSES for
Throat Chakra Flow:

*As with all poses listed here in Energy Types, please modify to suit
your own particular strength, flexibility and/or health challenges.*

EASY POSE (Sukhasana): With bottom on floor,
cross legs in a comfortable position, rest hands on
knees, palms facing up for more energy, facing down
to bring more relaxation. Lengthen spine by reaching crown towards the sky, open chest to allow for
full expansion of lungs.

NECK ROLLS: Lengthen the spine and on an inhale,
drop your chin to your chest. On exhale roll your
right ear to your right shoulder. Inhale and roll your
chin back to your chest. Exhale and roll your left ear
to your left shoulder. Inhale and roll the chin to the
chest. Repeat a few times back and forth.

SHOULDER SHRUGS: On an inhale, raise the
shoulders up towards the ears and as you exhale,
push them back opening the heart space and pressing shoulder blades towards one another, and relax-
ing down to a natural position.

AKASH MUDRA TWIST: Take the arms up to the sky and out
to the sides, palms up and coming into Akash Mudra, thumb and
middle fingers touching. As you exert slight pressure between the fingers, gently turn the body
from side to side, into Akash Mudra twist.
Continue this movement back and forth about 6
times and then come back to face center.

LION'S BREATH (Simhasana): Take a deep inhale
through the nose. Then simultaneously open your
mouth wide and stick out your tongue, curling it
downward toward the chin. Open the eyes wide, and
exhale the breath forcibly out through your mouth
making a "ha" sound. Repeat several times.

259

CRADLE ROCK (Apanasana): Draw your knees into your chest and wrap your arms around the upper part of your shins. Gently rock back and forth.

RECLINED COBBLER (Supta Badha Konasana):   Lie flat, feet flat on floor next to bottom, lower knees away from each other and bring soles of feet together. Elongate neck area by bringing shoulders down from ears. Hands rest alongside body, palms facing up.

SHOULDERSTAND: (Sarganvasana): Lying on floor with arms alongside the body, bend the knees bringing them towards the forehead. Place the hands under the hips to support the lower back and begin to lift the legs up, straightening them towards the sky. Support the weight of the body with the arms and the shoulders, placing very little weight in the head and neck. Relax the leg muscles and come into stillness. To come out, bend knees towards forehead, release hands and roll up to seated, or if proceeding to Plough Pose, allow legs to gently move towards floor.

PLOUGH: (Halasana): Using the ab muscles, lift the legs over the head until the toes touch the floor behind the head or just as far as they   gently choose to go OR if coming directly from Shoulderstand, as in this flow, just allow the legs to slowly fall towards the floor behind your head.   Support your lower back with your hands, elbows at shoulder width. Your hips should be aligned over the shoulders. (Don't force... just stretch to your own com-fort zone.)

STAFF POSE (Dandasana): Sit with legs stretched out in front of you, legs touching & parallel to floor. Sit up straight. Place hands next to hip area, spine long, thigh mus-cles engaged, heels slightly lifted off floor. Contract abs, open shoulders, elongate spine, crown rises towards ceiling and the gaze is gen-tly forward.

BEE'S BREATH (Brahmari): Place the thumbs over the ears and bring fingertips together at third eye, gently covering the eyes themselves. Then inhale through the nose, and when exhaling, hum. You will feel a mild buzzing within you (sounding much like the drone of a bee.) *Further clarification under Breathwork and Mudras.*

Throat Chakra Meditation

Whether you are seated or lying down, begin by bringing your attention to the moment... Allow any outside sounds to become distant as your awareness takes its place inside your being. Draw in a full inhalation and then let your exhale release any and all tension into the ground beneath you... big full inhales and exhales through the nose. As you begin to consciously ride the wave of the breath, let it cascade over you and through you, feeling it build, crest and blend back into the shore of your being.

Begin to practice Ujjayi breath, further expanding on this beautiful metaphor as the sound of the ocean massages and soothes the back of your throat space. Easy and flowing, a gentle 'ahhhh' sound as you inhale and exhale.

Now allow your attention to move to your root chakra... grounding... the fertile earth below you, a solid foundation on which to build. Breathe into this stability.

And now let your awareness move upward to your sacral chakra and the element of water and nourishment for your dreams. Imagine the seeds of creativity being planted in this fertile ground, nurtured and loved.

And further upward now into the brilliant yellow of your solar plexus, the sun within you. This golden glow bathes these seedlings of creation in its warmth and radiance.

And move still further now up into the realm of the heart, our seat of compassion. And here in a beautiful healing emerald light, the bud of a lotus blossom emerges, young and strong. With each breath, the petals open wider and wider... keep this breath pattern going until the lotus is fully in bloom.

This glorious flower rises up now into the broad blue expanse of your throat chakra - your seat of self-expression. Embrace this emerging creativity, filled with authenticity and the truth of YOU... And you are now ready to share your message, to share your gifts, to reveal them to the world. Continue to expand into this blue openness, like a wide open sky... and allow the echo deep within you to resonate into the world.

A wonderful light surrounds you as you bask in the knowing that you have made a difference. Continue to breathe and rest in this inner radiance and joy.

Namasté.

ENERGY TYPES

Third Eye Chakra Toolkit

Location: Between the Brows
Related Color: Indigo

When BALANCED...

Our sense of intuition is strong and guided, illuminating the path before us with the light of knowing.

When the SCALES ARE TIPPED...

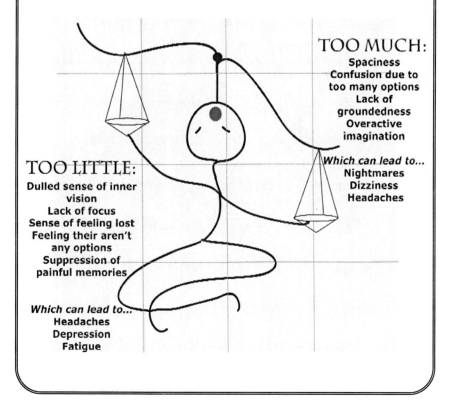

TOO MUCH:
Spaciness
Confusion due to too many options
Lack of groundedness
Overactive imagination

Which can lead to...
Nightmares
Dizziness
Headaches

TOO LITTLE:
Dulled sense of inner vision
Lack of focus
Sense of feeling lost
Feeling their aren't any options
Suppression of painful memories

Which can lead to...
Headaches
Depression
Fatigue

Still

allowing the pond of my mind
to grow still...
until an unbidden thought creates waves...

an internal wind blows fragments of words,
pieces of yesterday or tomorrow
churning until
i don't recognize them
and they meander to the shores
of past or future

breathe in the moment
reject the need to concentrate.
that just draws you
further from the truth
of what is

"what is" requires no thought.

ride the ripples of calm
to their destination
back to the starting point.
there you are.
still.

- *Maureen*

THIRD EYE CHAKRA
AJNA
("CENTER OF PERCEPTION AND COMMAND")

$\mathcal{O}$ur sixth energy field, the Third Eye, is located directly between the brows and honors our 'seat of intuition.' It is associated with the color of indigo. "Ajna" invites us to look deeply within to find the answers to our life questions. There exists an integral communication between the heart and our third eye because when we truly 'listen' to what our heart tells us, our intuition can never be wrong. We can then trust unquestioningly in the clarity that emerges from within this gateway of wisdom and inner knowing.

I find that there is also a strong correlation between the third eye and the root chakra: If we are overly immersed in our ideas and dreams, we may need grounding to realize them. And from the opposite perspective, if we are too rooted and feeling just plain stuck, we may need to open ourselves up to the gift of dreaming, imagining and trusting our 'inner knowing' to bring about manifestation.

Below are questions to ask yourself to determine your balance in the THIRD EYE CHAKRA:

You may be Third Eye Chakra deficient if you answer 'yes'
to any of the following:

* *Do I have difficulty envisioning my goals and sense of purpose?*
* *Is it hard for me to remember my dreams?*
* *Do I tend to question my 'gut feelings'?*
* *Am I feeling stuck in a stagnant routine?*

267

If you answered positively to any of these questions, it may be time to visit the THIRD EYE CHAKRA TOOLKIT and open the gates of intuition. Tuning into the HEART CHAKRA TOOLKIT will also allow your inner channels of guidance to shine a light on the true path of your life course.

You may be in Third Eye Chakra excess if you answer 'yes' to any of the following...

* *Am I experiencing confusion due to too many options?*
* *Do my friends jokingly call me space cadet and reel me back in to the earth plane?*
* *Am I having nightmares or anxiety-filled dreams?*
* *Am I having bouts of dizziness or difficulty separating dream life from reality?*

If you in the affirmative to any of these questions, you may need to anchor yourself and reconnect with earth energy through practices found in the ROOT CHAKRA TOOLKIT as well as truly listen to your heart by visiting the HEART CHAKRA TOOLKIT.

Third Eye Chakra: Breathwork & Mudras

APAN MUDRA: (ENERGY MUDRA) Bring the thumb, middle and ring fingers together to bring about a sense of serenity and inner balance. It opens us to the possibility of new beginnings and helps us 'see clearly' our path to future endeavors.

HAKINI MUDRA: (Hakini is god of the Third Eye Chakra) Bring all finger tips together forming a bridge between the hands. Place gentle pressure between the pads of the fingers. This mudra enhances our memory, concentration and ability to focus thus enabling our inner vision to be accessed with increased clarity.

KALESVARA MUDRA: (Dedicated to the diety Kalesvara, the Ruler of Time) This mudra calms the 'monkey mind' as well as feelings of frustration that can keep us feeling out of flow with our inner guide. Touch middle finger pads together pointing toward the sky, fold all other fingers inward (pinky, ring and index) thumbs touching pointing towards your heart.

Third Eye Chakra Intention:
Working with the Third Eye Chakra flow will bring awareness to your naturally intuitive nature and open the doors of imagination. Allow your focus to rest in the indigo light between the brows and enhance the guidance emerging from within.

Affirmation for Third Eye Chakra:
I am guided by the light of inner vision and intuitively trust the path before me.

THIRD EYE CHAKRA FLOW

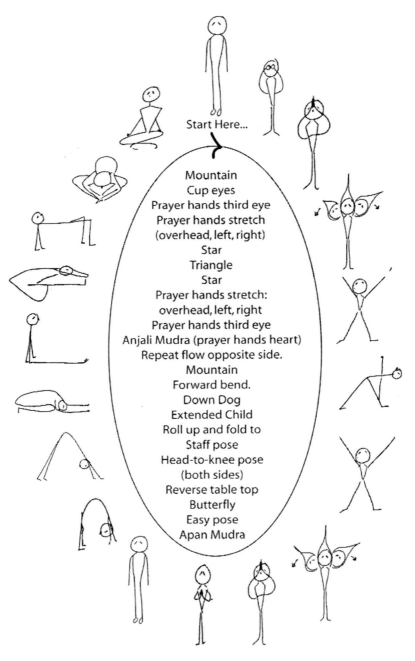

Start Here...

Mountain
Cup eyes
Prayer hands third eye
Prayer hands stretch
(overhead, left, right)
Star
Triangle
Star
Prayer hands stretch:
overhead, left, right
Prayer hands third eye
Anjali Mudra (prayer hands heart)
Repeat flow opposite side.
Mountain
Forward bend.
Down Dog
Extended Child
Roll up and fold to
Staff pose
Head-to-knee pose
(both sides)
Reverse table top
Butterfly
Easy pose
Apan Mudra

Description of YOGA POSES for
Third Eye Chakra Flow:

As with all poses listed here in Energy Types, please modify to suit your own particular strength, flexibility and/or health challenges.

MOUNTAIN (Tadasana): Stand erect with feet hip width apart (or if your balance is good you can have feet touching). Hands loose at sides, spine lengthened, shoulders up, back and down, eyes gaze forward. Feel the earth beneath your feet.

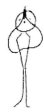

CUP EYES: Still in mountain pose, rub hands to create warmth. Cup your eyes and draw breath into the third eye space.

PRAYER HANDS (Anjali Mudra) **at THIRD EYE**: Bring hands together and rest them on third eye space, allowing the backs of the thumbs to exert gentle pressure.

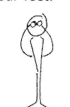

PRAYER HANDS STRETCH: Stretch hands in prayer pose towards sky, elongating spine, feet grounded. Then bend and stretch to the right, breathe into the side ribs. Bend and stretch to the left, breathe into side ribs. Back to center. (In flow, repeat in reverse direction i.e. right then left).

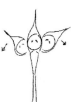

STAR POSE: From mountain with hands still elevated, step right foot out to the side (approx. 3 ft. or to your comfort zone). Open arms hands to the sky and glance towards the heavens.

TRIANGLE (Trikonasana): With feet spread 3-4 feet apart, turn your right foot 90 degrees to the right and your left foot about 45 degrees inward. Bring both arms parallel to floor and stretch your right arm out to the side, folding and bringing your right hand to rest against inside of your right calf (again placement will depend on flexibility. Attempt to remain in a straight plane). Now raise left hand to the sky, palm facing forward and turn to gaze at your hand. Repeat flow on opposite side.

FORWARD BEND (Uttanasana): Start in mountain. Take hands up to sky, then exhale, bend at the waist, sweeping arms down. Legs can be straight or knees slightly bent if hams feel stiff. Keep weight toward the front of your feet to avoid leaning backwards. Relax your neck, allowing the crown of your head to reach toward the ground.

DOWNWARD FACING DOG (Adho Mukha Svanasana): Curl toes under and push back, raising hips towards sky and straightening legs. Position hands shoulder width apart, feet hip width apart. Weight evenly distributed front and back. Lower heels towards floor. Allow your head to gently hang between arms, chest towards earth.

EXTENDED CHILD: Sit on your feet, knees comfortably separated, straighten your back and lift up, stretch arms out in front of you and relax your neck, resting head between arms.

STAFF POSE (Dandasana): Sit with legs stretched out in front of you, parallel to floor. Sit up straight. Place hands next to hip area, spine long, thigh muscles engaged, heels slightly lifted off floor. Contract abs, open shoulders, elongate spine, crown towards ceiling & gaze

HEAD-TO-KNEE FORWARD BEND (Janu Sirsasana): From staff pose, high on sitbones, bend left knee bringing sole of foot to inside of right thigh. Inhale, reach up with both arms creating more length in spine. Exhale and fold forward from base of hip joints. The hands come down to rest on either side of right thigh as you continue to lengthen front of the torso from pelvis to breastbone. (You can also use a strap looped around foot to prevent rounding of spine.)

REVERSE TABLE TOP: In staff pose, bring hands back by bottom, fingertips pointing towards hips. Bend knees & ground feet. Inhale, lengthen spine, on exhale draw belly in and lift hips up. Keep nose parallel to ceiling, extending out through crown so that spine & neck are in one straight line. On inhale continue to lengthen, on exhale, allow bottom to sink back to floor.

BUTTERFLY (Yin Yoga style): With weight on front edge of sitting bones, bend knees, press soles of feet together, let your legs drop out like butterfly wings. Take heels at least a foot away from hips. Cup toes or hold ankles bending forward from hips to your own comfort zone, relax upper spine and let it round. Rest your headand neck.

EASY POSE (Sukhasana): With bottom on floor, cross legs in a comfortable position, rest hands on knees, palms facing up for more energy, facing down to bring more relaxation. Lengthen spine by reaching crown towards the sky, open chest to allow for full expansion of lungs.

Third Eye Chakra Meditation

This is a meditation designed to access the gifts that Ajna, our third eye chakra, offers us as our innate intuitive advisor. We will be using two different Mudras (or symbolic positioning of our hands) to enhance the spiritual reflection. First we will activate Apan Mudra - which literally translated from Sanskrit means "energy mudra." It contains the power of shaping visions of the future and a springtime-like feel of welcoming new beginnings. Join your thumb, ring and middle fingers, and extend the index and pinky fingers, with palms facing up. The second Mudra we will engage is called the Kalesvara Mudra (which is dedicated to the diety Kalesvara, the ruler of time.) This mudra calms the 'monkey mind' (mind chatter) as well as feelings of frustration that can keep us feeling 'out of flow.' The calmer and clearer we become, our minds like pools of tranquil, clear, reflective water, the easier it is to tap into new insights and welcome the guidance that propels us in joyful, purposeful direction. To practice this mudra, bring middle finger pads together pointing toward the sky, all other fingers folded inward (pinky, ring and index), and thumbs touching pointing towards your heart.

Make sure that you will have a few minutes to disconnect from any outside distractions so that you can fully embrace the magic of the moment. Whether you are seated on the floor in Sukhasana /cross-legged or in a chair, take care that your spine is elongated, knees level if crosslegged, feet grounded if in a chair.... We will begin in Apan Mudra (thumb, middle and ring fingers touching) representing an open mind, new beginnings, like a seedling planted in the soil of your intuition. Allow your breath and focus to become as a gentle rain ushering growth, manifestation, and realization of your desires.

Breathe now into this expansion... breathe into the indigo light glowing softly between your brows... your internal knowing. Take five long inhales and exhales ... completing each cycle with awareness.

Continue to focus on the newness of your path... and as you do, bring your hands into Kalesvara Mudra - (middle finger pads together pointing toward the sky, other fingers folded inward, thumbs touching pointing towards heart.) Let your breath become even longer, deeper, slower.... Bring special attention to the flow, to the space between the breaths at the top of the inhale and bottom of the exhale... Full... belly... breaths...

As you merge into this stillness, a scene opens before you, projected from Ajna... your third eye space. You are walking along a beautiful forest path, the warm sunshine filtering through the trees warming your face, your back... As you continue along your way, you notice someone in the distance walking towards you, a Being dressed all in white, almost glowing in the beams of sunlight. You keep advancing towards one another and as you come closer, you notice that he (she) is carrying something. When you are near enough to look into one another's eyes, your Messenger holds out a scrolled piece of white paper with a gold ribbon tied around it and places it lovingly in your hands. As you take the scroll, the Being dissolves into a fine white light, leaving only the rays of the sun where they once stood. You walk over to the stump of a large tree and settle yourself on the smooth, warm surface. Slowly and tenderly, you remove the gold ribbon.... You unroll the scroll... And there in beautiful script is a message... Words of love and light and direction meant just for you. You close your eyes and continue to breathe into these words that are both a revelation as well as achingly familiar.

Continue to breathe long, deep breaths. Lower your hands back into Apan Mudra and allow the essence of your message to blend into the indigo light of Ajna.

May you know love. May you know joy. May you know calm... as you surrender to being both filled and emptied along your expanding path of Divine purpose, trusting in the guidance within you.

Namasté.

Crown Chakra Toolkit

Location: Top of Head
Related Color(s): Lavender, White

When BALANCED...

We celebrate our connection with the Divine, recognizing UNITY CONSCIOUSNESS.

The current of life force energy (Prana) flows with ease and we realize an inner freedom and peace.

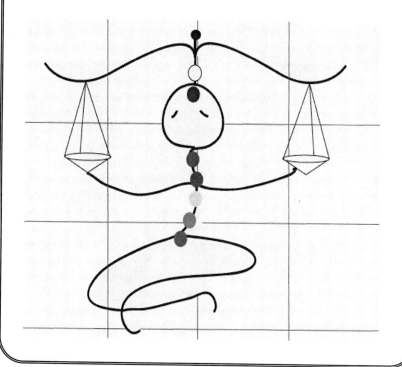

celestial bliss

i can hold
the moon
in one hand
and fly across oceans.

ride the waves
of falling stars
as they dance
through the heavens.

stare the universe
straight in the eye
and say
"pardon the intrusion,
but is this my stop?
I'm looking for
celestial bliss
and my map
led
me
here."

- *Maureen*

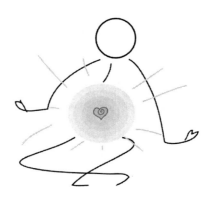

CROWN CHAKRA
(SAHASRARA) - Connection to the Divine

*W*hen first teaching yoga, I would proceed week after week, honoring the different energy fields, beginning with the root chakra, working our way up to the third eye. The cycle would then begin anew, returning to Muladhara (root). I intentionally bypassed Sahasrara, figuring, how can I teach a class that might seemingly offer the rewards of an open crown chakra and possible enlightenment? Will my students expect to leave class walking two feet above the ground in a state of Nirvana?

Then one day, a good friend who joined me on a regular basis voiced her desire to indeed be including this energy field in the line-up. So, the answer to the question of how to best honor Sahasrara became a flow that would honor ALL the chakras and in this way, pay homage to the beauty of *all* energy fields. The goal of our practice was to bring about a balance of Yin and Yang, equating to overall peace and joy within.

For this particular chakra, I have chosen to offer what I call "Qi-Yoga-ng" uniting QiGong with Yoga-like flows. QiGong has been practiced in China for over 5000 years and is "a discipline that combines mental concentration, breathing technique, and body movements to activate and cultivate our 'vital energy.'"[5] Thus the pairing of the two seemed ideal for the crown chakra.

But first, let us look at some breathwork and mudras that can enhance your practice when paying tribute to this field.

Crown Chakra: Breathwork & Mudras

ALTERNATE NOSTRIL BREATHING: (Nadi Shodhana) 'Nadi" in Sanskrit means 'little river' and in this case refers to the channels through which energy flows. 'Shodhana' means purification so this practice will bring about a clearing of the energy pathways. It purifies and lends balance to the energy on both sides of our body, and hence, all chakras.

To practice this form of pranayama, fold the middle two fingers of the right hand into the palm and extend the other three. We begin the process breathing into the left side: Use your thumb to first close the right nostril and inhale through the left nostril for the count of four. Then close the left nostril with your right ring finger and at the same time remove your thumb from the right nostril, and exhale through this nostril for the count of four. This completes a half round. Now with the left nostril closed with ring finger, inhale through the right nostril to the count of four. Close the right nostril with your right thumb and exhale through the left nostril to the count of four. This completes one full round.

Continue this for at least eight cycles and work your way up to twelve.

PRANA MUDRA: (LIFE/ENERGY MUDRA) Bring the tips of the thumbs, ring and pinky fingers together, extending the other two. Practicing this mudra will bring a sense of calm, balance and increased vitality to your entire being. (Also excellent for revving up the root chakra!)

DHYANI MUDRA: (MEDITATION MUDRA) Form an 'empty bowl' by placing your left hand inside the right hand, palms facing up allow the thumbs to gently touch and lay your hands in your lap. This is a simple pose that you can use to allow the rains of grace to 'fill your bowl' (though in actuality we are never empty...) You can practice this whenever you are meditating and quiet the 'monkey mind' thus allowing new fresh energy to flow into your being and give you the guidance that most suits your current situation.

Crown Chakra Intention:
To honor all of our beautiful chakras while
breathing into the healing light, balance
and peace within.

Affirmation for Crown Chakra:
I open myself to a higher, deeper power and
trust my connection with the Divine.

Description of Qi-YOGA-ng POSES for
Crown Chakra Flow:

As with all poses listed here in Energy Types, please modify to suit your own particular strength, flexibility and/or health challenges.

While I have suggested a certain number of repetitions for each of the flows, feel free to practice any of the moves for several minutes, especially if you are seeking healing and balance in a particular chakra.

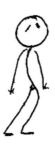

OPENING POSTURE: Bounce lightly on your feet from the balls to the heels, finding an easy stable stance. Your toes point forward, your feet are a bit wider than shoulder width, your knees slightly bent, your spine long and straight, your eyes closed or looking softly before you. Your tongue gently touches the roof of your mouth as this activates the front and back energy channels of the body. Your hands hang loosely at your sides, fingers open to allow the flow of energy. Remain in this posture for a few breaths, coming into the silence within and affirming your connection with the Universe.

ROOT CHAKRA: Draw your hands out and up overhead and start to shake them, building energy up inside your whole hand and fingers. Keep shaking through two inhales and then on the second exhale, slowly lower them down the front of the body, palms facing down, to hip level, feeling the energy sink back down towards the earth. Repeat 3 more times.

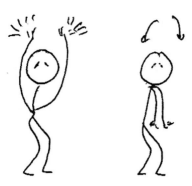

SACRAL CHAKRA: Move the hands in front of your sacral chakra area and hold them approximately 6-8 inches apart. Picture a ball of light between them and begin breathing into this light . Start to gently pulse your hands back and forth, but don't allow them to touch. Feel the energy building between them. Now begin to form an 'infinity flow' taking the ball of light in the shape of a sideways figure 8. Roll from side to side and slightly shift your weight as well from side to side as you move with the flow. Repeat several times.

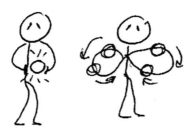

SOLAR PLEXUS CHAKRA: Now bring the ball of light back in front of your body and raise it to solar plexus level. As you lift the ball up towards the sky, pivot to your left, coming up on the back toe, hands raised to the sky. Then sweep the ball back down to center and pivot to the right. As you flow side to side, bring awareness to your internal organs (liver, stomach, spleen, gallbladder) being bathed in healing light. Continue back and forth three more times and then return to center, raising the ball of light straight up to the heavens.

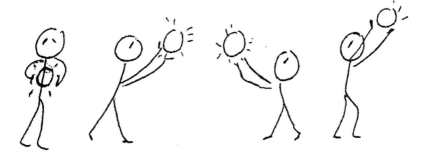

HEART CHAKRA: Now release the ball of light to the heavens and lower the arms out to the sides, coming into Chin Mudra (index finger and thumb joined). As you inhale, raise the arms up overhead and gently touch the tips of the fingers to the crown, forming a heart shape with the arms. On the exhale, with palms facing you, lower the hands down to heart level and then turn the palms out, pushing them into the space before you, and then opening them out to the sides, spreading heart radiance all around you. Come once more into Chin Mudra, arms open at your sides. Repeat this flow 3 more times.

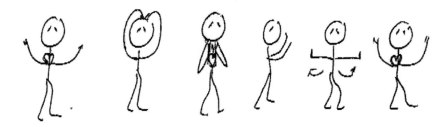

THROAT CHAKRA: Now draw the hands together in front of the throat chakra in Padme Mudra (Lotus Mudra) with palms (at wrist), pinkies and thumbs touching, all other fingers extended. Inhale, and on the exhale take the lotus out into the space in front of you, sharing your gifts of creativity with the world. Then inhale and continue to raise the lotus up to the sky, open the arms out to the sides, exhale sweeping them out and down, coming together at the sacral chakra. Then again inhale, raising them back up to Padme Mudra at the throat space. Repeat 3 more times.

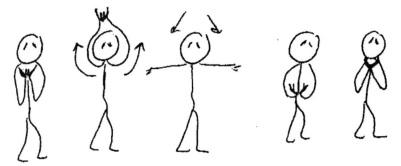

THIRD EYE CHAKRA: Take the hands now in Anjali Mudra (prayer hands) up to the third eye space between the brows and breathe into the indigo light. On an inhale, raise them up above your head and on the exhale, sweep the arms out to the sides and gently fold forward bringing the fingertips to the earth. On the next inhale, rise up to standing, head coming last to avoid dizziness and bring the hands once more to the third eye chakra in Anjali Mudra. Repeat 3 more times.

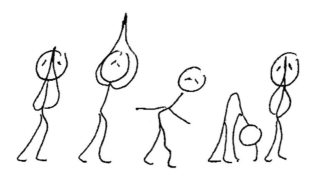

CROWN CHAKRA: Raise both hands up to the heavens and with open fingers, begin to make circles with wrists, blending the energy of Yin and Yang (female and male energies.) Keep breathing and circling, picturing all the energy channels in the body open and filled with light. Then lower the arms out the sides, bringing the hands into Prana Mudra, the life force mudra and allow yourself to settle into a peaceful state preparing for the crown chakra meditation.

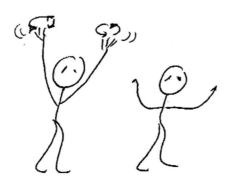

Crown Chakra Meditation

Release the past, do not worry about the future... Bring all of your awareness into this moment. Let your breath flow in through your crown and gently down your entire body and find yourself in a loving space where you have nothing to do but BE. Prepare now to do a chakra cleansing to bring all of your energy fields into perfect balance.

Become aware of your posture. If you are seated, sense the earth under your feet, lengthen your spine towards the heavens, hands lay gentle upon your lap. If you are lying down, feel the length of your body secure and grounded, your weight releasing into the earth beneath you more and more with every breath.

Relax your jaw, your neck and gently close your eyes. Take a couple of great big inhales through the nose and exhale through the mouth, releasing any tension that may have built up within your body. Then come back to a nice even breath through the nose with continued awareness on the present.

Now picture a ball of radiant white light that is hovering just above your crown chakra. As you breathe into this light, draw it down in through your crown and allow it to float down your neck, your full spine until it comes to rest at the root chakra at the base of your spine where it mingles with a beautiful red light. Breathe into this red light and affirm, "I am grounded, protected and all of my needs are met."

Continue to breathe into the ball of light and allow it to journey upward until it rests in your sacral chakra and merges into a vibrant orange. As you breathe into this orange light, I want you to affirm,

286

"I flow easily and fluidly with the current of my life, without resistance."

Now the ball of light floats even further upward until it reaches the solar plexus chakra and blends into a radiant yellow, like the sun within you. As you breathe into this yellow light, affirm, "I claim my personal power and move forward with courage and confidence."

The journey continues as the ball of light moves up into the heart chakra, our seat of compassion, where it first meets with a beautiful gold light, as our heart emanates the color gold, and then blends with a brilliant emerald green. Breathe into this green light and affirm, "I connect with harmony and peace as I give and receive love with ease."

The ball of light now moves up still further into the throat chakra and a brilliant blue. As you breathe into the blue light, our seat of communication, affirm, "I clearly speak my inner truth and express my creativity joyfully to the outside world."

And now the ball of light journeys still further upward until it comes to the space between your brows, where it merges with an indigo light in the third eye chakra, our seat of intuition. As you breathe into this light, affirm, "I am lovingly guided by an inner knowing and visualize my perfect path with clarity and ease."

The ball of light leaves the third eye chakra and makes its way first through a lavender light that then becomes the brilliant white light of the crown chakra. As you breathe into this radiance, affirm,

"I open myself to a higher, deeper power and trust completely my connection to the Divine."

And now this white light disperses and rains over you and through you, illuminating every cell and fiber of your being. Radiant now, pefectly aligned. Breathe into this balance knowing all is indeed well.

Namasté.

Chapter 5
TAKING AIM:
Affirmation, Intention & Motion

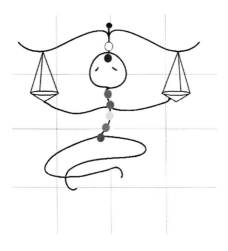

TAKING AIM: Affirmation, Intention & Motion

The following flows are not specifically type-related, but offered as a means of promoting balance in dealing with some general life issues or needs that anyone could be experiencing.

TAKING AIM refers to movement flows that incorporate:
* Affirmation (Thought)
* Intention (Feeling) &
* Motion (Energy)

I feel that the combination of these three elements truly has the potential to assist in the manifestation of what it is you desire more of in your life, be that more freedom, more love, more joy, more abundance, more direction, better health...

In the following pages, we will explore three separate flows. The first will assist in the releasing of what is no longer serving you to make room for the new. The second is a healing flow that will direct loving energy within your own body and spirit, or to another person, pet, plant, or any other being in your life. And finally, the third will address the art of surrendering to our Divine Purpose.

We will be combining affirmations with motion as well as mudras to intensify the intention behind the movement.

Let's begin by taking a closer look at the use of affirmations and how we can make them even more potent in our lives. Saying an affirmation is most powerful when stated in the present tense as well as in a positive format. We can also greatly enhance the beneficial effects by repeating them from 3 different perspectives. The first person activates your own truth, the second and third person statements deepen the impact as if from an outside source. For example:

* I am in perfect vibrational harmony with boundless joy.
  (affirming what you know to be true)
* YOU are in perfect vibrational harmony with boundless joy.
  (verification from 'outside source')
* SHE (or HE) is in perfect vibrational harmony with boundless joy.
  (verification from an observer standpoint)

"Feeling" your life wish from this 3-dimensional stance adds greatly to the depth of the experience.

On that note, FEELING is key in working with affirmations in general and that is where INTENTION comes in. If you are saying you desire boundless joy while FEELING worried and concerned, you are sending out mixed signals. This is also where the MOTION becomes key. Not only are you bringing your focus into the moment, you are allowing the energy around your intention to flow more freely and at the same time removing blockages to the desired outcome.

So now let's look at some areas where you can practice TAKING AIM.

RELEASING THE OLD, EMBRACING THE NEW:

When letting go of something in your life that is no longer serving you, we must first look with GRATITUDE at whatever we wish to release, whether we see the blessing in it at this point or not... (Blessings can indeed come in strange packages.) We then open ourselves to the JOY of the newness for which we are making space.

Begin this exercise with an affirmation:
I now choose to release the old and embrace the new.
You now choose to release the old and embrace the new.
She/he is now chooses to release the old and embrace the new.

The movement flow goes like this:

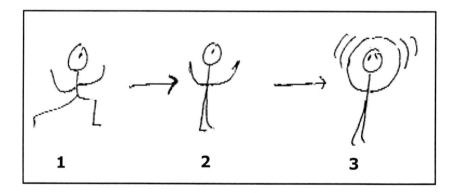

1   **2**   **3**

1) Stand in an elevated lunge, right foot back, left foot forward, knee bent to 90 degrees directly over ankle. The arms are out the sides, palms up in Prithivi/Earth Mudra (thumb and ring finger touching). Bring awareness to the grounding of the forward foot and the antipated 'lifting off' of the back foot. The affirmation and intention are as follows: **IN GRATITUDE, I RELEASE THE OLD.**

2) Now step the back foot forward to meet the other, coming into mountain pose, but with arms still out to sides, palms up moving into an Apan /Energy Mudra (thumb, ring and middle fingers touching (open to newness and growth) and the affirmation and intention become: **IN JOY, I EMBRACE THE NEW.**

3) Now repeat on opposite side, stepping left foot back into elevated lunge, right foot forward, in Prithivi Mudra. **IN GRATITUDE, I RELEASE THE OLD.** Step forward to mountain and Apan Mudra: **IN JOY, I EMBRACE THE NEW.**

When complete, flow the arms in three big, fluid circles to allow the energy of your intention to move freely into manifestation.

This entire exercise can be repeated several times. If you are able to practice this in a meadow, on a beach or anywhere that is expansive, you can keep the momentum going by continuing to move forward. This will further enhance the idea of letting go and moving on.

PERFECT HEALTH / INFINITY FLOW HEALING EXERCISE

This is a flow to bring healing either to yourself or to anyone else, be it a person, pet, plant or any sentient being desiring optimum health and balance. It's always important to ask permission if you are sending healing energy to someone else, allowing the object of the intention to accept whatever they deem necessary. Always remember, too, the innate perfection that resides within each one of us, no matter the 'outside' appearance.

Begin this exercise with an affirmation:
I now choose perfect health.
You now choose perfect health.
She/he now chooses perfect health.

The movement flow goes like this:

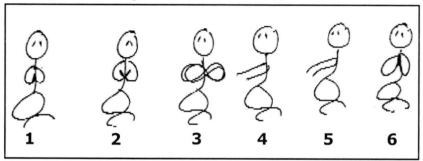

1) Begin with hands on heart and draw your inhale down through the crown of your head, filling your heart space with the 'breath of healing' and love. As you exhale send this healing and love into your hands. Repeat several times.

2) Bring the hands into Lotus Mudra at the heart, allowing this healing and love to blossom.

3) With your hands a few inches in front of your heart space, palms facing out, begin to move them in an 'infinity flow' (figure 8 motion) to build and intensify the strength of the healing and love. At this time, if you are practicing healing on yourself, begin to focus on the perfection of whatever area to which you are sending this healing. If you are practicing on someone else, whether they are right there with you or in a remote location, ask for their permission to send this healing energy to them and give them the option of embracing whatever or however much of this energy they wish to receive.

4) Now open your hands palms facing up. 'Feel' and see the energy flowing out from your fingertips in brilliant streams of light to the object of your healing. Remain in this position until it feels complete.

5) Next, turn your palms to face the earth to seal in the healing love.

6) Bring your hands back to your heart in Anjali Mudra (prayer hands) giving gratitude for the healing that has taken place and for being a conduit for the endless current of Universal Love.

SURRENDERING TO OUR DIVINE PURPOSE

This flow honors love, joy, connectedness to all, the opening of our being to the rains of grace, the emptying of our being to what doesn't serve and in completion, the surrender to our Divine Purpose.

Begin this exercise with an affirmation:
I willingly surrender to my Divine Purpose.
You willingly surrender to your Divine Purpose.
She/he willingly surrenders to her/his Divine Purpose.

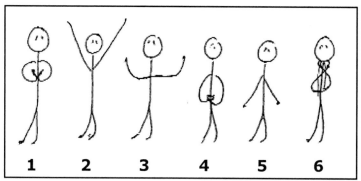

1) Begin with hands on heart, the seat of compassion, in Lotus Mudra. **Affirm with loving intention: I AM LOVE.**

2) Take the vibration of love up through the light of the crown chakra, raising the arms up to the sky, palms open. **Affirm with loving intention: I AM JOY.**

3) Lower the arms out to your sides, bringing hands into Chin Mudra (thumb and index finger touching). **Affirm with loving intention: I AM CONNECTED (to all sentient beings).**

4) Lower the hands down in front of the lower belly, housing the left hand in the right, thumbs touching into Dhyani Mudra, the mudra of contemplation, like a bowl that is filling up with the rains of grace. **Affirm with loving intention: I AM FILLED.**

5) Next, release the hands down to the sides, palms facing Mother Earth. **Affirm with loving intention: I AM EMPTIED.**

6) Then bring your right hand to the left shoulder, your left hand to the right shoulder in a self-embrace, lowering the head towards the heart. **Affirm with loving intention: I SURRENDER TO MY DIVINE PURPOSE.**

ENERGY TYPES

CHAPTER 6

In Closing...

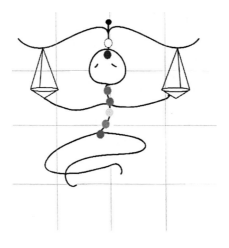

DANCE, CHILD, DANCE

I looked up to God, 'cause I felt kinda low-
Needed some guidance on which way to go...
Thought it was all being left up to chance-
The answer I heard, was "Dance,Child, Dance."

Your life is a dance, each day and each night,
Reach for the heavens, soar like a kite!
Let your energy flow with the wind,
And your path will find YOU, again and again.

I pondered the message, it seemed so near...
Just let go and the road would be clear?
Find that place between 'trying and not'-
Where dreams become real and the dance is taught.

So now I dance, sometimes fast, sometimes slow.
The sound of my heartbeat says which way to go-
Those elusive answers, once so out of reach
Are now dancing round me- It's my turn to teach.

Your life is a dance, each day and each night,
Reach for the heavens, soar like a kite!
Let your energy flow with the wind,
And your path will find YOU, again and again.

Follow your heart.

- Maureen

In Closing...

You may have recognized various references to 'dancing' throughout the book. This is because whether we are waltzing through life, finding ourselves in need of executing a side-step, or even choosing to 'sit one out,' we are here on this earth to be joyful! Challenging times will present themselves, to be sure, but if we can maintain a peaceful, balanced inner landscape, the moves will prove much easier to perform, step by step.

My dearest wish is that the information found within these pages has and will continue to offer you tangible support, heightened self-understanding, and increased communication with others. May *Energy Types* be a roadmap that will guide you in honoring the beauty that is YOU.

Keep trusting in that magic.

Namasté,
Maureen

ENERGY TYPES

Acknowledgements

The encounters we experience in our everyday lives are gifts and lessons whether they be a shared glance in passing or a relationship that spans decades. I would need to include an additional chapter, should I begin to thank all those who have touched my life and added to the messages and information found within *Energy Types*.

But now I *would* like to offer special gratitude to the teachers who have blessed my life thus far, as well as some sensational 'soul sisters' who are sharing the road.

Heartfelt gratitude to William (Bill) Jeffries, my colleague and dear friend whose belief in me regarding my work with the MBTI® was a sturdy platform on which to build. I am honored to know you and hope to continue walking the path with you that leads others to increased self-understanding and communication. (Erfolg kennt keine Grenzen.)

Deepest appreciation to Juliet Jivanti, my wonderful 'sister' and yoga teacher... Meeting Juliet rekindled the spark within me regarding my love of yoga and meditation that led to these roads converging. What a blessing you are in my life.

Sincere gratitude to Barefoot Doctor (Stephen Russell), who has opened my heart to the beautiful experience of the Tao. I so look forward to exploring the Warrior path with you for a long time to come. Your teachings are a gift not only to me, but to the multitudes and I'm honored to have you in my life. CHI!

To my beautiful soul sisters: Ellen, Faith, Audrey, Crystal, Nari, Stacey, Adele and my dear Yoginis who join me each week for our Chakra Yoga Flow. Your support means the world!

As always thanks to my treasured 4-leggeds (Francesca, Bo, Jack, Nick, Simba and Bianco Nove) who surround me with their love as I write and pace and stretch and breathe (and sometimes swear). They share it all!

I would like to also thank Hay House for the guidance you have offered as well as the friendships I have made through listening to your inspirational radio show.

And last but certainly not least, a deep bow to John Lennon whose energy and love is always guiding me. ("Any time at all...")

Notes

Chapter 1
1. Dr. Deborah Tannen, *You Just Don't Understand*, p. 52, Ballantine Books, New York, 1990
2. Sue Monk Kidd, *When the Heart Waits*, quoting C. G. Jung, p. 51, Harper Collins, 2006
3. C. G. Jung, *Memories, Dreams, Reflections*, p. 395, Vintage Books Edition, 1989

Chapter 2
1. Anodea Judith, *Chakra Balancing Workbook*, p 2, Sounds True, Sebastool. CA, 2003
2. David R. Hamilton, Ph.D., *How Your Mind Can Heal Your Body*, p. 170, Hay House, Inc., 2010
3. Gertrud Hirschi, *Mudras - Yoga in your Hands*, p. 2, Red Wheel/Weiser, 2000

Chapter 4
1. Gertrud Hirschi, *Mudras - Yoga in your Hands*, p. 62, Red Wheel/Weiser, 2000
2. Institute of Heart Math, www.heartmath.org
3. Melody Beattie, *Language of Letting Go - Daily Meditations For Codependents*, Harper Collins, 1990
4. Institute for Applied Meditation/University of the Heart, www.iamheart.org
5. Chunyi Lin, *Spring Forest QiGong for Health*, Learning Strategies Corporation, Minnesota

ENERGY TYPES

Suggested Reading...

In the books recommended below you will find further in-depth information on the MBTI® as well as chakras, energy, healing and manifestation.

On Personality Type / MBTI®:

STILL TRUE TO TYPE by William C. Jeffries: A comprehensive look at the most frequently asked questions about completing and interpreting the MBTI®. Excellent resource for the practitioner as well as individuals interested in further exploring the benefits of this instrument, offered from one of the world's top authorities on Type.

TYPE TALK or How to Determine Your Personality and Change Your Life by Otto Kroeger and Janet Thuesen: A superb introduction to the MBTI® with in-depth explanations of individual preferences as well as detailed profiles. Also filled with very entertaining anecdotes and stories. Should be part of every 'Type Lovers' library.

GIFTS DIFFERING by Isabel Briggs Myers with Peter B. Myers: Could be considered the original 'bible' of Type. Written by the creator of the MBTI®, it offers a detailed look at understanding personality differences, perceptions and conclusions and the importance of integrating this knowledge into your daily life.

PLEASE UNDERSTAND ME - Character & Temperament Types by David Keirsey and Marilyn Bates: A look at how knowing just two letters of your MBTI® type can reveal information on your living, loving and learning styles.

On Chakras:

CHAKRA BALANCING WORKBOOK by *Anodea Judith:* A beautifully written overview of our energy fields including extensive information on all seven chakras. Highly recommended for those wishing to deepen their knowledge of our energy fields.

ANATOMY OF THE SPIRIT - The Seven Stages of Power and Healing by *Caroline Myss:* This book presents Dr. Myss's look at three spiritual traditions - the Hindu chakras, the Christian sacraments and the Kabbalah's Tree of Life - expressing the seven stages we each go through in our quest for spiritual maturity. A wonderful overview of the chakras, including correlations with mental, emotional and physical issues associated with each field.

On Healing Energy and Manifestation:

From Barefoot Doctor (Stephen Russell):
MANIFESTO - How to Get What You Want Without Trying & RETURN OF THE URBAN WARRIOR- High-speed Sprituality for People on the Run: Based on Taoist philosophy, each of these books offers techniques designed to streamline your life experience through visualization, relaxation, meditation and self-healing techniques. Superb writing style (and often laugh-out-loud funny as well...)

HOW YOUR MIND CAN HEAL YOUR BODY by *Dr. David R. Hamilton, Ph.D.:* Explores the influence of our thoughts on our body and how we can alter the state of our health through visualization. An outstanding look at the merging of science and belief.

WHEN THE HEART WAITS- Spiritual Direction for Life's Sacred Questions *by Sue Monk Kidd:* A touching tale of spiritual awakening and moving from a place of gripping pain to a place of joy. For anyone and everyone looking to embrace life's challenges and come out not only stronger, but whole and complete on the other side, this is an utterly beautiful (true) story of spiritual transformation.

And so very many more... I'm deeply grateful to the authors who have touched my life in myriads of ways!

LaVergne, TN USA
30 October 2010
202887LV00003B/1/P

About the Author...

Maureen has been working with the Myers-Briggs Type Indicator® since 1990 when she received her certification with Otto Kroeger Associates in Fairfax, Virginia. Since that time, she has greatly enjoyed working with individuals and businesses, helping people better understand their own personal styles as well as enhancing their communication skills with others in their lives.

Fitness has also been a long-time love of hers (including many years of distance running and triathloning) and the introduction of yoga into her life was key in bridging the gap between the physical and the spiritual. She completed her yoga teacher training in 2007 allowing her to share her love of the practice with others.

Learning, teaching and sharing are key components that keep the joy flowing. And now she hopes to contribute to the well-being of many more folks through the 'convergence of these two roads.'

P.S. No recap would be complete in describing the life of Maureen Kelly if her love of animals wasn't mentioned. (She's a little bit nuts that way. So bring on the ENFJ soapbox!)

To contact Maureen, email her at sagebutterfly2@comcast.net or visit her website: www.energy-types.net.